STUDY GUIDE
FOR
MEMMLER'S

The Human Body
in Health
& Disease

Barbara Janson Cohen, BA, MSEd
Assistant Professor
Delaware Community College
Media, Pennsylvania

Dena Lin Wood, RN, MS
Staff Nurse
VNA Care
Glendale, California

STUDY GUIDE FOR MEMMLER'S

The Human Body
in Health
& Disease

9*th Edition*

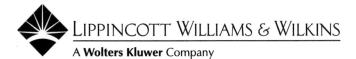

LIPPINCOTT WILLIAMS & WILKINS
A **Wolters Kluwer** Company
Philadelphia • Baltimore • New York • London
Buenos Aires • Hong Kong • Sydney • Tokyo

Acquisitions Editors: Margaret M. Biblis, John Butler
Editorial Assistant: Amy Amico
Managing Editor: Barbara Ryalls
Senior Production Manager: Helen Ewan
Production Coordinator: Mike Carcel
Art Director: Carolyn O'Brien

9th Edition

9 8 7

Library of Congress Cataloging-in-Publication Data

ISBN: 0-7817-2111-3

Care has been taken to confirm the accuracy of the information presented and to describe generally accepted practices. However, the authors, editors, and publisher are not responsible for errors or omissions or for any consequences from application of the information in this book and make no warranty, express or implied, with respect to the contents of the publication.

The authors, editors and publisher have exerted every effort to ensure that drug selection and dosage set forth in this text are in accordance with current recommendations and practice at the time of publication. However, in view of ongoing research, changes in government regulations, and the constant flow of information relating to drug therapy and drug reactions, the reader is urged to check the package insert for each drug for any change in indications and dosage and for added warnings and precautions. This is particularly important when the recommended agent is a new or infrequently employed drug.

Some drugs and medical devices presented in this publication have Food and Drug Administration (FDA) clearance for limited used in restricted research settings. It is the responsibility of the health care provider to ascertain the FDA status of each drug or device planned for use in their clinical practice.

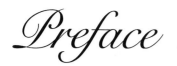

Preface

Study Guide for Memmler's The Human Body in Health & Disease, ninth edition, assists the beginning student to learn basic information required in the health occupations. Though it will be more effective when used in conjunction with the ninth edition of *The Human Body in Health and Disease,* the Study Guide may also be used to supplement other textbooks on basic anatomy and physiology.

The questions in this edition reflect revisions and updating of the text. The labeling exercises are taken from the all-new illustrations designed for the book. The "Practical Applications" section of each chapter uses clinical situations to test understanding of a subject. Comparing the normal with the abnormal helps a student to gain some understanding of disease prevention and health maintenance.

The exercises are planned to help in student learning, not merely to test knowledge. A certain amount of repetition has been purposely incorporated as a means of reinforcement. Matching questions require the student to write out complete answers, giving practice in spelling as well as recognition of terms. Other question formats include multiple choice, completion, true–false, and short essays. The true–false questions must be corrected if they are false. The essay answers provided are examples of suitable responses, but other presentations of the material are acceptable.

All answers to the *Study Guide* questions are in the *Instructor's Manual* that accompanies the text.

Contents

Unit I

THE BODY AS A WHOLE

1

Organization of the Human Body

I. Overview

Living things are organized from simple to complex levels. The simplest living form is the *cell*, the basic unit of life. Specialized cells are grouped into *tissues*, which, in turn, are combined to form *organs;* these organs form *systems*, which work together to maintain the body.

The systems include the integumentary system, the body's covering; the skeletal system, the framework of the body; the muscular system, which moves the bones; the nervous system, the central control system that includes the organs of special sense; the endocrine system, which produces the regulatory hormones; the circulatory system, consisting of the heart, blood vessels, and lymphatic vessels that transport vital substances; the respiratory system, which adds oxygen to the blood and removes carbon dioxide; the digestive system, which converts raw food materials into products usable by cells; the urinary system, which removes wastes and excess water; and the reproductive system, by which new individuals of the species are produced.

All the cellular reactions that sustain life together make up *metabolism,* which can be divided into *catabolism* and *anabolism.* In catabolism, complex substances, such as the nutrients from food, are broken down into smaller molecules with the release of energy. This energy is stored in the compound *ATP* (adenosine triphosphate) for use by the cells. In anabolism, simple compounds are built into substances needed for cell activities.

All the systems work together to maintain a state of balance or *homeostasis.* The main mechanism for maintaining homeostasis is negative feedback, by which the state of the body is the signal to keep conditions within set limits.

Study of the body requires knowledge of directional terms to locate parts and to relate various parts to each other. Several *planes of division* represent different directions in which cuts can be made through the body. Separation of the body into areas and regions, together with the use of the special terminology for directions and locations, makes it possible to describe an area within the human body with great accuracy.

The large internal spaces of the body are the **cavities,** in which various organs are located. The *dorsal cavity* is subdivided into the cranial cavity and the spinal cavity (canal). The *ventral cavity* is subdivided into the thoracic and abdomino-pelvic cavities. Imaginary lines are used to divide the abdomen into regions for study and diagnosis.

The metric system is used for all scientific measurements. This system is easy to use because it is based on multiples of 10.

II. Topics for Review

A. Studies of the body
B. Body systems
C. Body processes
D. Directions in the body
E. Body cavities
    1. Dorsal cavity
    2. Ventral cavity
       a. Regions of the abdomen
F. The metric system

III. Matching Exercises

Matching only within each group, write the answers in the spaces provided.

Group A

tissue	organ	cell
system	anatomy	pathology
physiology		

1. The basic unit of life   *cell*

2. The study of body structure   *anatomy*

3. A specialized group of cells   *tissue*

4. The study of disease   *pathology*

5. A group of organs functioning together for the same
   general purpose   *system*

6. The study of how the body functions   *physiology*

7. A combination of tissues that function together   *organ*

Group B

umbilicus	diaphragm	epigastric
thoracic	transverse	lateral
frontal		

1. A plane that divides the body into superior and inferior parts *transverse*

2. A directional term that means away from the midline
   (toward the side)   _____

3. A plane that divides the body into anterior and posterior parts _____

4. Another name for the navel   *umbilicus*

5. Term describing the central region of the abdomen just
   below the breast bone   *epigastric*

6. The muscular partition between the two main ventral
   body cavities   _____

7. A term that describes the uppermost (chest) portion of the
   ventral body cavity   _____

Group C

| sagittal | proximal | posterior |
| caudal | cranial | horizontal |

1. A term that indicates a location toward the back   _____

2. A term that means closer to the origin of a part   _____

3. A plane that divides the body into left and right parts   _____

4. A word that means nearer to the sacral (lowermost) region of the spinal cord   _____

5. A plane of division that also is described as a transverse or cross section   _____

6. A word that means nearer to the head   *cranial*

Group D

respiratory system   integumentary system   skeletal system
endocrine system   reproductive system   urinary system

1. The system that includes the sex organs   *reproductive*

2. The system made up of the bones and joints   *skeletal*

3. The system of scattered organs that produce hormones   *endocrine*

4. Another name for the excretory system   *urinary*

5. The system made up of the lungs and the passages leading to and from the lungs   *respirtory*

6. The system that includes the hair, nails, and skin   *integumentary*

IV. Multiple Choice

Select the best answer and write the letter of your choice in the blank.

1. Another name for a coronal plane is   1. _____

   a. distal
   b. horizontal
   c. frontal
   d. transverse
   e. sagittal

2. The term *ventral* means   2. _____

   a. toward the belly surface
   b. posterior
   c. in the dorsal body cavity
   d. farther from the origin of a structure
   e. nearer to the back

3. Anabolism produces   3. ____*a*____

   a. simple compounds from more complex compounds
   b. carbon dioxide
   c. energy
   d. complex materials needed for body functions
   e. digested foods

4. Fluids located outside the cells are described as

    a. lateral
    b. intracellular
    c. superior
    d. extracellular
    e. frontal

4. _____d_____

5. A system that controls and coordinates the body is the

    a. circulatory system
    b. nervous system
    c. urinary system
    d. digestive system
    e. skeletal system

5. _____b_____

6. The cavity below the abdominal cavity is the

    a. dorsal cavity
    b. frontal cavity
    c. thoracic cavity
    d. cranial cavity
    e. pelvic cavity

6. _____

7. A plane that divides the body into upper and lower parts is called a

    a. transverse plane
    b. frontal plane
    c. midsagittal plane
    d. superior plane
    e. sagittal plane

7. _____

V. Labeling

For each of the following illustrations, write the name or names of each labeled part on the numbered lines.

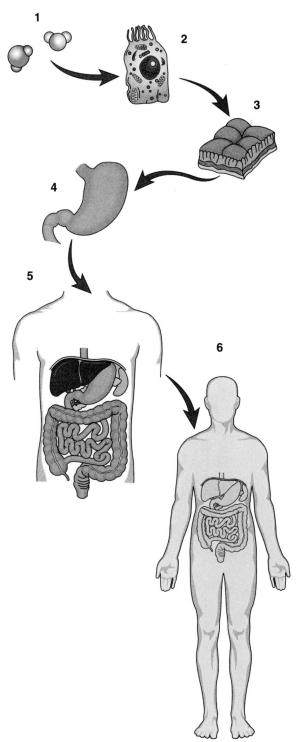

1. <u>chemicals</u>
2. <u>cells</u>
3. <u>tissue</u>
4. <u>organ</u>
5. <u>system</u>
6. <u>whole system</u>

Levels of organization

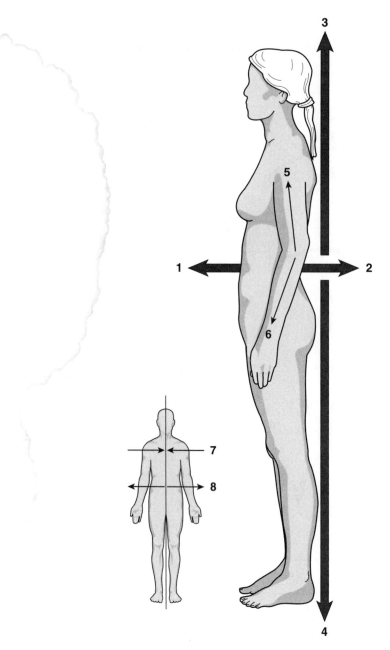

Directional terms

1. ventral, anterior
2. Posterior, dorsal
3. Superior
4. inferior
5. Proximal
6. distal
7. midline
8. lateral

1 **2** **3**

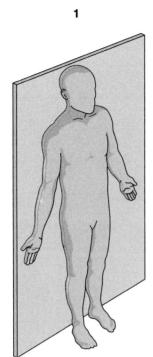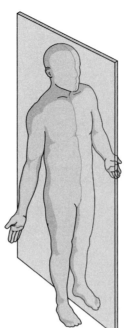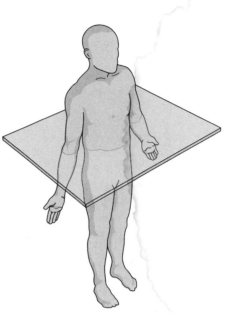

Planes of division

1. _Frontal_

2. _saggital_

3. _transverse_

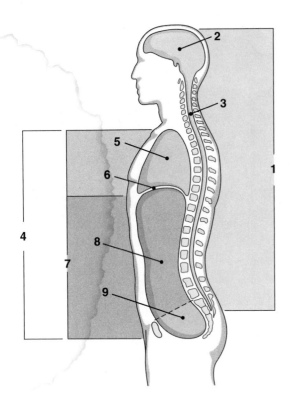

Side view of body cavities

1. _Dorsal_
2. _Cranial_
3. _Spinal_
4. _ventral_
5. _Thoratic_
6. _diagraphm_
7. _abdominopelvic_
8. _abdominal_
9. _Pelvic_

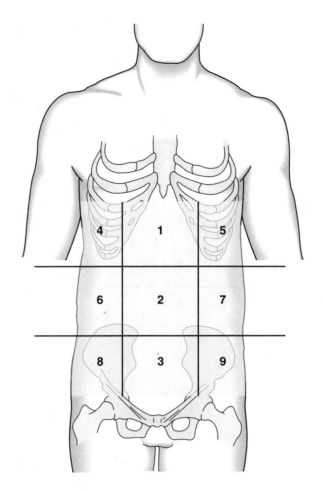

Regions of the abdomen

1. Epigastric
2. umbilicus
3. hypogastric
4. R hypochondric
5. (L) hypochondric

6. Right lumbar
7. (L) lumbar
8. (R) ttie lliac
9. (L) ittie llic

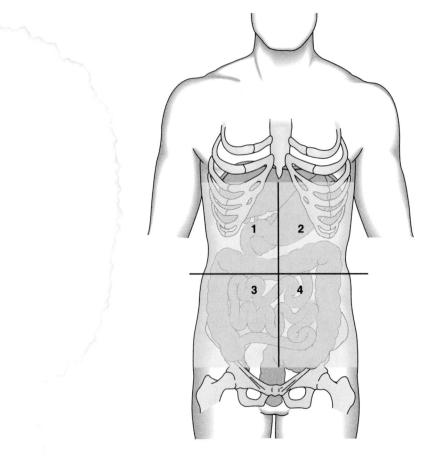

Quadrants of the abdomen

1. _R^ quadrant_

2. _L^ quadrant_

3. _R L quadrant_

4. _L L quadrant_

VI. True–False

For each question, write T for true or F for false in the blank to the left of each number. If a statement is false, correct it by replacing the underlined term and write the correct statement in the blanks below the question.

___T___ 1. In <u>catabolism</u>, nutrients are broken down into simpler compounds.

_____

_____

___F___ 2. Another term for dorsal is <u>anterior</u>.

_posterior_____

_____

I   3. The term <u>caudal</u> means toward the head.

inferior

_____

T   4. The word <u>medial</u> indicates nearness to the midsagittal plane.

_____

_____

F   5. The term <u>proximal</u> means away from the point of origin.

near.

_____

VII. Completion Exercise

Group A

Write the word or phrase that correctly completes each sentence.

1. Regions and directions in the body are described according to the position in which the body is upright, with the palms facing forward. This is called the   _anatomic_

2. A specialized group of cells make up a(n)   _tissue_

3. All the chemical reactions that sustain life make up   _____

4. Negative feedback is a mechanism for maintaining an internal state of balance known as   _hemostasis_

5. The elongated canal that contains the spinal cord is known as the   _____

6. The main compound that stores energy in the cell is   _ATP_

7. The midline plane that divides the body into right and left halves is the   _sagittal_

8. The space that encloses the brain and spinal cord forms a continuous cavity called the   _cranial_

9. The ventral body cavity includes an upper space containing the lungs, the heart, and the large blood vessels, which is called the   _Thoracic_

10. The space that houses the brain is the _____

11. The plane that divides the body into anterior and posterior parts is the _____Frontal_____

12. The ventral body cavity that contains the stomach, most of the intestine, the liver, and the spleen is the _____

13. The abdomen may be subdivided into nine regions, including three along the midline. The uppermost of these midline areas is the _____abdominal_____

14. The abdomen may be divided into four regions, each of which is called a(n) _____quadrant_____

15. The main large ventral body cavities are separated from each other by a muscular partition called the _____diaphragm_____

Group B

Write the word that correctly completes each sentence about the metric system.

1. The standard unit for measurement of length is the _____meteric_____

2. The number of grams in a kilogram is _____1000_____

3. The number of centimeters in an inch is _____100_____

4. The standard unit for measurement of volume, slightly greater than a quart, is a(n) _____liter_____

5. The number of milliliters in 0.5 liter is _____

VIII. Practical Applications

Study each discussion. Then write the appropriate word or phrase in the space provided.

Group A

1. The gallbladder is located just below the liver. The directional term that describes the position of the gallbladder with regard to the liver is _____

2. The kidneys are located behind the other abdominal organs. This position may be described as _____

3. The wrist is located farther from the shoulder than is the elbow. The term that describes the position of the wrist with regard to the elbow is _____

4. The entrance to the stomach is nearest the point of origin or beginning of the stomach, so this part is said to be

_____

5. The ears are located away from the midsagittal plane or toward the side, so they are described as being

_____

6. The head of the pancreas is nearer the midsagittal plane than its tail portion, so the head part is more

_____

7. The diaphragm is above the abdominal organs; it may be described as

_____

8. Ms. B was experiencing pain in the area of her left ovary. Her physician ordered an ultrasound study of which quadrant of the abdomen?

_____

Group B

On the ward for the care of postoperative patients, you are asked to study the following cases and to answer the questions based on the nine divisions of the abdomen.

1. Mr. A had an appendectomy. The appendix is in the lower right side of the abdomen. In which of the nine abdominal regions is it located?

_____

2. Ms. D had a history of gallstones. The operation to remove these stones involved the upper right part of the abdominal cavity. Which of the nine abdominal regions is this?

_____

3. Ms. C was injured in an automobile accident. In addition to a number of fractures, she suffered a ruptured urinary bladder. The region involved, in the lower midline part of the abdomen, was the

_____

4. Mr. B required an extensive exploratory operation that necessitated incision through the navel. This portion of the abdomen is in what region?

_____

Group C

The triage nurse in the Emergency Room was showing a group of students how she assessed patients with disorders in different body systems.

1. Each client was assessed for changes in the color of the outer covering of the body. The outer covering is called the skin, which is part of the

_____

2. One person had been injured in a fall, producing an injury to the framework of the body. This framework is known as the

_____

3. A young man who had been practicing tennis reported that after lunging for a ball he had a sharp pain in the calf of his leg. Now he was limping. The nurse suspected a tear to structures belonging to the

_____

4. A middle-aged woman was brought in with loss of ability to move the right side of her body. The nurse felt that a blood clot in the brain was producing the symptoms. The brain is part of the controlling system known as the

_____

5. A young woman reported bulging eyes; pounding, fast heart rate; and much sweating. The nurse suspected overactivity of a hormone-producing structure. The glands that produce hormones make up the

_____

6. An older man was brought in by ambulance with severe pain in the chest. It was suspected that there was a disorder of the heart, the organ that pumps blood through the

_____

7. A man complaining of pain in the abdomen and vomiting blood was brought in by his family. A problem was suspected in the system responsible for taking in food and converting it to usable products. This system is the

_____

8. A young woman asked to see the doctor about pain in the hypogastric region of her abdomen. She reported a need to empty her bladder frequently. The bladder is part of the

_____

9. A young pregnant woman in labor requested admission to the hospital to deliver her baby. The production of offspring is the function of the

_____

IX. Short Essays

1. Define *metabolism* and describe the two phases of metabolism.

_____

_____

_____

2. Explain homeostasis and how negative feedback works to maintain homeostasis.

_____

_____

_____

3. Explain why specialized terms are needed to indicate different positions and directions within the body.

_____

_____

_____

2

Chemistry, Matter, and Life

I. Overview

Chemistry is the physical science that deals with the composition of matter. To appreciate the importance of chemistry in the field of health, it is necessary to know about elements, atoms, molecules, compounds, and mixtures. An *element* is a substance consisting of just one type of atom. Although exceedingly small particles, atoms possess a definite structure: the *nucleus* contains *protons* and *neutrons,* and surrounding the nucleus are the *electrons.*

Union of two or more atoms produces a *molecule;* the atoms in the molecule may be alike (as in the oxygen molecule) or different (sodium chloride, for example). In the latter case, the substance is called a *compound.* A combination of compounds, each of which retains its separate properties, is a *mixture.* Mixtures include solutions, such as salt water, and suspensions. In the body, chemical compounds are constantly being formed, altered, broken down, and recombined into other substances.

Water is a vital substance composed of hydrogen and oxygen. It makes up more than half of the body and is needed as a solvent and a transport medium. Hydrogen, oxygen, carbon, and nitrogen are the elements that constitute about 96% of living matter, whereas calcium, sodium, potassium, phosphorus, sulfur, chlorine, and magnesium account for most of the remaining 4%.

Isotopes (forms of elements) that give off radiation are said to be *radioactive.* Because they can penetrate tissues and can be followed in the body, they are useful in diagnosis. Radioactive substances also have the ability to destroy tissues and can be used in the treatment of many types of cancer.

Proteins, carbohydrates, and lipids are the organic compounds characteristic of living organisms. An important group of proteins are the *enzymes,* which function as catalysts in metabolism.

II.   Topics for Review

A. Elements and atoms
B. Molecules and compounds
C. Water, solutions, and suspensions
D. Chemical bonds
E. pH and buffers
F. Radioactivity
G. Organic compounds

III.   Matching Exercises

Matching only within each group, write the answers in the spaces provided.

Group A

nucleus   pharmacology   element
chemistry   atom   organic

1. The science that deals with the composition of all matter   _____

2. The smallest complete unit of matter   _____

3. Term for the chemical compounds that characterize
   living things   _____

4. The study of all aspects of drugs   _____

5. A substance composed of one type of atom

_____

6. The part of the atom containing most of its mass including protons and neutrons

_____

Group B

isotopes   radioactivity   neutrons
molecule   compounds   protons
mixture   electrons

1. The noncharged particles within the atomic nucleus

_____

2. A combination of different substances, each of which remains intact and retains its properties

_____

3. The positively charged particles inside the atomic nucleus

_____

4. Elements existing in forms that are alike in their chemical reactions but that differ in weight

_____

5. The negatively charged particles outside the atomic nucleus

_____

6. The emission (giving off) of rays from disintegrating isotopes

_____

7. The unit formed by the union of two or more atoms

_____

8. Substances that result from the union of two or more different atoms

_____

Group C

cations   carbohydrates   acid
electrolytes   anions   water
pH   proteins   buffer

1. Negatively charged ions

_____

2. The universal solvent

_____

3. A substance that donates a hydrogen ion to another substance

_____

4. The category of organic compounds that includes simple sugars and starches

_____

5. Compounds that form ions when in solution

_____

6. Positively charged ions

_____

7. A measure of the acidity of a solution

_____

8. A substance that helps to maintain a stable hydrogen ion concentration in a solution

_____

9. Organic compounds that contain nitrogen in addition to carbon, oxygen, and hydrogen

_____

Group D

elements	amino acid	phospholipids
suspension	colloidal suspension	covalent
atomic number	solute	

1. Nitrogen, carbon, hydrogen, and oxygen, for example

_____

2. Term for a chemical bond formed by the sharing of electrons

_____

3. A feature that identifies each element

_____

4. A building block of proteins

_____

5. A mixture in which substances will settle out unless the mixture is shaken

_____

6. The group of lipids that contains phosphorus in addition to carbon, hydrogen, and oxygen

_____

7. Cytoplasm and blood plasma are examples of this type of mixture

_____

8. A substance that is dissolved in another substance

_____

Group E

ionic	carbon	neutral
radioactivity	lipid	enzyme
neutrons		

1. Another name for a fat

_____

2. Particles that vary in number in different isotopes

_____

3. The element contained in all organic compounds

_____

4. A type of protein that acts as a catalyst in metabolic reactions

_____

5. The type of bond that forms an electrolyte

_____

6. Term that describes a pH of 7.0

_____

7. Cancer therapy includes the use of needles, seeds, or tubes containing isotopes that have this property

_____

IV. Multiple Choice

Select the best answer and write the letter of your choice in the blank.

1. Which of the following is *not* a common chemical element
   in the body?

   a. nitrogen
   b. carbon
   c. oxygen
   d. copper
   e. hydrogen

   1. _____

2. Which of the following statements is *not* true of water?

   a. It is a compound.
   b. It can dissolve many different substances.
   c. It is organic.
   d. It is stable at ordinary temperatures.
   e. It contains hydrogen and oxygen.

   2. _____

3. A mixture that is not a solution but does not separate because the
   particles in the mixture are so small is a(n)

   a. colloidal suspension
   b. solvent
   c. radioactive isotope
   d. true solution
   e. enzyme

   3. _____

4. Which of the following statements is *not* true of electrolytes?

   a. They conduct an electrical current in solution.
   b. They separate into charged particles in solution.
   c. They are compounds.
   d. They are found in body fluids.
   e. They are insoluble in water.

   4. _____

5. The pH scale ranges from

   a. 5 to 10
   b. 0 to 14
   c. 10 to 20
   d. 3 to 6
   e. 0 to 20

   5. _____

6. Which of the following statements is *not* true of enzymes?   6. _____

   a. Their names usually end in the suffix *-ase.*
   b. Their shape is important in reactions.
   c. They are used up in reactions.
   d. They are altered by extreme temperatures.
   e. They speed up the rate of a reaction.

V. Labeling

For each of the following illustrations, write the name or names of each labeled part on the numbered lines.

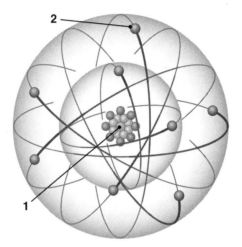

Oxygen atom

1. _____   2. _____

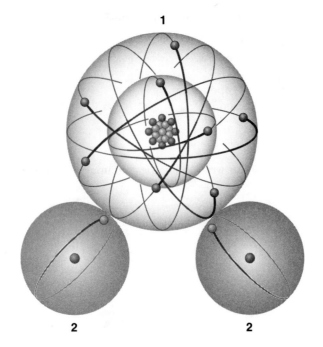

1

2   **2**

Molecule of water

1. _____   2. _____

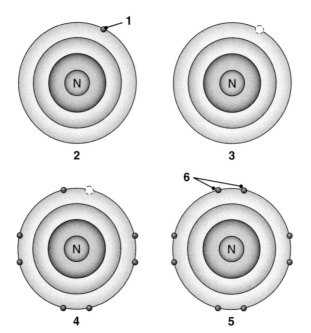

Formation of sodium cation and chlorine anion

1. _____   4. _____

2. _____   5. _____

3. _____   6. _____

VI. True–False

For each question, write T for true or F for false in the blank to the left of each number. If a statement is false, correct it by replacing the underlined term and write the correct statement in the blanks below the question.

_____ 1. The charged particles in the nucleus of an atom are called <u>neutrons</u>.

_____

_____

_____ 2. The first energy level of an atom can hold <u>eight</u> electrons.

_____

_____

_____ 3. An atom that normally loses electrons to attain a complete outer energy level is called a <u>metal</u>.

_____

_____

_____ 4. The smallest unit of a compound is a <u>molecule</u>.

_____

_____

_____ 5. A positively charged ion is an <u>anion</u>.

_____

_____

_____ 6. A <u>covalent</u> bond is one formed by the sharing of electrons.

_____

_____

_____ 7. A pH of <u>10.0</u> is neutral.

_____

_____

_____ 8. A substance that can accept a hydrogen ion is an <u>acid</u>.

_____

_____

_____ 9. Fats are examples of <u>lipids</u>.

_____

_____

_____ 10. Monosaccharides are the building blocks of <u>carbohydrates</u>.

_____

_____

VII. Completion Exercise

Write the word or phrase that correctly completes each sentence.

1. The four elements that make up about 96% of living cells are oxygen, carbon, and hydrogen plus _____

2. Many people keep a shaker of salt on the table. Salt is an example of a combination of two different elements. Such a combination is called a(n) _____

3. The element that is the basis of organic chemistry is _____

4. The smallest particle of a compound that has all the properties of that compound is a(n) _____

5. Salt water is a mixture in which one substance is dissolved in another and remains evenly distributed. This type of mixture is a(n) _____

6. If an electron is added to or removed from an atom, it becomes a charged particle, also known as a(n) _____

7. Metabolic reactions require organic catalysts called _____

8. Many essential body activities depend on certain compounds that form ions when in solution. Such compounds are called _____

9. The name given to a chemical system that prevents changes in hydrogen ion concentration is

_____

VIII. Practical Applications

Study each discussion. Then write the appropriate word or phrase in the space provided. The following medical tests are based on principles of chemistry and physics.

1. Mr. B complained of shortness of breath. Several studies were done including a visible tracing of the electric currents produced by his heart muscle. Such a record is called a(n)

_____

2. Joan, age 4, was brought to the clinic by her mother because she experienced attacks of fainting and unconsciousness. As an aid in diagnosis, a graphic record of her brain's electric current was obtained. This brain wave record is called a(n)

_____

3. A routine test done on Ms. J showed glucose in her urine, an abnormal finding. Glucose and other sugars belong to a group of organic compounds classified as

_____

4. Mr. K's urinalysis showed the presence of albumin. Albumin is an example of compounds found in the body that contain nitrogen, carbon, hydrogen, and oxygen. These compounds are classified as

_____

5. Mrs. L, age 72, was brought to the clinic with symptoms of decreased function of many systems. Her history revealed poor fluid intake for several weeks. Her symptoms were due to a shortage of the most abundant compound in the body, which is

_____

6. Mrs. L had blood drawn to check on certain common elements found in body fluids. The blood was to be tested for concentrations of the elements sodium, potassium, chloride, and others. These elements are parts of salts that separate into ions in solution and are referred to as

_____

7. The blood test for Mrs. L included measurement of blood urea nitrogen (BUN). Urea is a by-product of protein metabolism. The building blocks of proteins are called

_____

8. Allen, age 10, fell while riding his bicycle. He had pain and swelling of the right arm. His examination included a procedure in which rays penetrate body tissues to produce an image on a photographic plate. The rays used for this purpose are called

_____

IX. Short Essays

1. Describe the structure of an atom.

   _____

   _____

   _____

2. What properties make water an ideal medium for living cells?

   _____

   _____

   _____

3. Why is carbon the basis of organic chemistry?

   _____

   _____

   _____

4. Why is the shape of an enzyme important in its function?

   _____

   _____

   _____

3 Cells and Their Functions

I. Overview

The cell is the basic unit of life; all life activities result from the activities of cells. The study of cells began with the invention of the light microscope and has continued with the development of electron microscopes. Cell functions are carried out by specialized structures within the cell called *organelles.* These include the nucleus, ribosomes, mitochondria, Golgi apparatus, and endoplasmic reticulum (ER).

An important cell function is the manufacture of *proteins,* including enzymes (organic catalysts). Protein manufacture is carried out by the ribosomes in the cytoplasm according to information coded in the deoxyribonucleic acid (DNA) of the nucleus. DNA also is involved in the process of cell division or *mitosis.* Before cell division can occur, the DNA must double itself so each daughter cell produced by mitosis will have exactly the same kind and amount of DNA as the parent cell.

The plasma (cell) membrane is important in regulating what enters and leaves the cell. Some substances can pass through the membrane by *diffusion,* which is simply the movement of molecules from an area where they are in higher concentration to an area where they are in lower concentration. The diffusion of water through the cell membrane is termed *osmosis.* Because water can diffuse very easily across the membrane, cells must be kept in solutions that have the same concentrations as the cell fluid. If the cell is placed in a solution of higher concentration (a hypertonic solution), it will shrink; in a solution of lower concentration (a hypotonic solution), it will swell and may burst. The cell membrane can also selectively move substances into or out of the cell by *active transport,* a process that requires energy (ATP) and transporters. Large particles and droplets of fluid are taken in by the processes of *phagocytosis* and *pinocytosis.*

When cells undergo a genetic change, or mutation, so that they multiply out of control, the result is a tumor. A tumor that spreads to other parts of the body is termed *cancer*. Risk factors that influence the development of cancer include heredity, chemicals (carcinogens), ionizing radiation, physical irritation, diet, and certain viruses.

II. Topics for Review

A. Microscopes
B. Cell structure
C. Protein synthesis
D. Cell division (mitosis)
E. Movement of materials across the plasma membrane
F. Cells and cancer

III. Matching Exercises

Matching only within each group, write the answers in the spaces provided.

Group A

active transport   mitosis   diffusion
osmosis   isotonic   filtration

1. The passage of solutions through a membrane as a result of mechanical force

Filtration

2. Term for a solution that has the same concentration of molecules as the fluids within the cell

Isotonic

3. The process by which water molecules diffuse through the cell membrane

osmosis

4. The process of body cell division

mitosis

5. The spread of molecules throughout an area

diffusion

6. The process by which the cell uses energy to move substances across the membrane

active transport

Group B

plasma membrane   lysosomes   nucleolus
cilia   ribosomes   endoplasmic reticulum
mitochondria   flagellum

1. Small bodies in the cytoplasm that act in the manufacture of proteins

Ribosomes

2. A system of membranes throughout the cell

endoplasmic reticulum

3. A small body within the nucleus

nucleolus

4. Small hairlike projections from the cell used to create movement around the cell

cilia

5. The organelles that convert energy into ATP

mitochondria

6. The outer covering of the cell

plasma membrane

7. Small bodies in the cell that contain digestive enzymes

lysosomes

8. A long, whiplike extension used in cell locomotion

flagellum

Group C

DNA   nucleotides   centriole
proteins   genes   RNA
cholesterol   ATP

1. The organelle that is active in cell division

Centriole

2. The hereditary factors in the cell

genes

3. The chemical in the nucleus that makes up the chromosomes

4. The substances manufactured according to the DNA code

proteins

5. Building blocks of nucleic acids

6. The main energy compound of the cell

7. The nucleic acid that carries information from the nucleus to the ribosomes

_____

8. A substance that strengthens the plasma membrane

_____

Group D

pinocytosis   osmotic pressure   carcinogen
hypotonic   hypertonic   prophase
mutation

1. Term for a solution that is less concentrated than the fluid within the cell

hypotonic

2. The force that draws water into a solution

osmotic pressur

3. The process by which a cell takes in droplets

pinocytosis

4. Any cancer-causing chemical

carcinogen

5. Term for a solution with a salt concentration greater than 0.9%

hypertonic

6. The first stage of mitosis

prophase

7. Any change in the genetic material of a cell

mutation

IV. Multiple Choice

Select the best answer and write the letter of your choice in the blank.

1. Which of the following statements is *not* true of the plasma membrane?

   a. It protects the cell.
   b. It keeps nutrients out.
   c. It is composed mainly of lipids and proteins.
   d. It is semipermeable.
   e. It regulates what enters and leaves the cell.

1. *D*

2. Which of the following statements is *not* true of mitosis?

   a. The original cell produces two identical daughter cells.
   b. It follows duplication of DNA in the nucleus.
   c. It occurs at the same rate in all cells.
   d. It involves the centrioles and a spindle.
   e. It results in equal division of the chromosomes.

2. *C*

3. The stage of mitosis during which the chromosomes line up across the spindle is called

   a. metaphase
   b. anaphase
   c. prophase
   d. telophase
   e. none of the above

3. *a*

4. The substance that moves most rapidly through the cell membrane is   4. ___d___

    a. glucose
    b. lipid
    c. DNA
    d. water
    e. sucrose

5. Which of the following are required for active transport?   5. ___b___

    a. vesicles and cilia
    b. transporters and ATP
    c. mitosis and diffusion
    d. osmotic pressure and centrioles
    e. osmosis and lysosomes

6. Which of the following solutions is isotonic for body cells?   6. ___e___

    a. 5% salt
    b. distilled water
    c. 10% glucose
    d. 10% dextrose
    e. 0.9% salt

V. Labeling

For each of the following illustrations, write the name or names of each labeled part on the numbered lines.

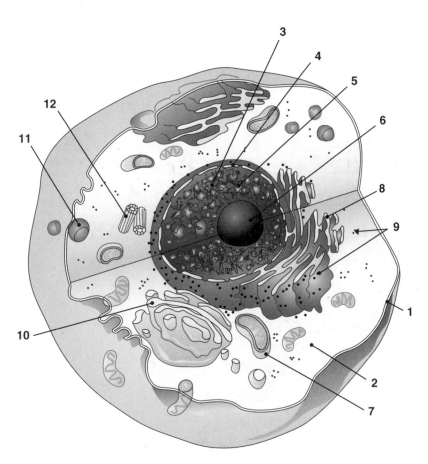

Typical animal cell showing the main organelles

1. Plasma membrane
2. Cytoplasm
3. Nucleus
4. Nuclear membrane
5. Genetic material (DNA)
6. Nucleolus
7. Mitochondrion
8. Endoplasmic reticulum
9. Ribosomes
10. Golgi apparatus
11. lysomes
12. Centriole

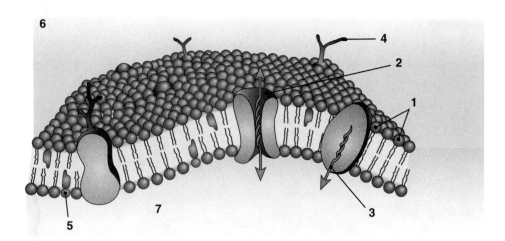

Structure of the plasma membrane

1. Phospholipids
2. Membrane Protein
3. Protien channel
4. Carbohydrate
5. Cholesterol
6. Extracellular Fluid
7. Cytoplasm

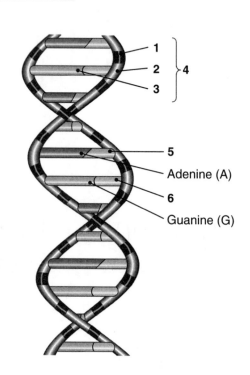

Adenine (A)

Guanine (G)

Basic structure of a DNA molecule

1. Phosphate unit
2. Sugar unit
3. nitrogen base
4. nucleotide
5. Thymine (T)
6. Cytosine (c)

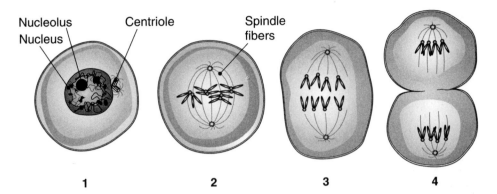

Nucleolus   Centriole   Spindle fibers
Nucleus

1   2   3   4

Stages of mitosis

1. ___Prophase___   3. ___anaphase___
2. ___metaphase___   4. ___telophase___

(type of solution)

3   5   7

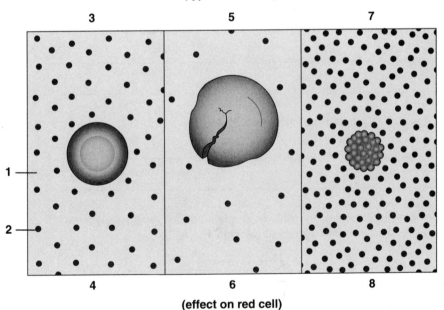

4   6   8

(effect on red cell)

Osmosis

1. ___water___   5. ___Hypotonic___
2. ___Solute___   6. ___Swollen/ruptured___
3. ___Normal Isotonic___   7. ___Hypertonic___
4. ___normal___   8. ___Shrunken red___

37

VI. True–False

For each question, write T for true or F for false in the blank to the left of each number. If a statement is false, correct it by replacing the underlined term and write the correct statement in the blanks below the question.

___F___ 1. The ribosomes are made of <u>DNA</u>.

_____

___F___ 2. A solution that is more concentrated than the intracellular fluid is described as <u>hypotonic</u>.

___less concentrated than intracellular___
___fluid___

___T___ 3. A 5% dextrose solution is <u>isotonic</u> for body cells.

_____

___T___ 4. A long, whiplike extension from the cell is called a <u>flagellum</u>.

_____

___T___ 5. A cell placed in a hypotonic solution will <u>swell</u>.

_____

___T___ 6. In the <u>anaphase</u> stage of mitosis, the duplicated chromosomes separate and move toward opposite ends of the cell.

_____

_____

VII. Completion Exercise

Write the word or phrase that correctly completes each sentence.

1. The metric unit that is commonly used to measure cells is the _____

2. The substance that fills the cell and holds the cell contents is the

cytoplasm

3. The process of cell division is called

mitosis

4. Small structures within a cell that perform special functions are called

_____

5. The control center of the cell, which contains the chromosomes, is the

nucleus

6. The cell membrane uses energy to move materials from low concentration to a higher concentration (opposite to the direction they would normally flow by diffusion). The membrane therefore is described as

active transport

7. Chromosomes are composed mainly of

_____

8. The chromosomes duplicate during the period between mitoses, which is called

interphase

9. Cells engulf large particles by the process of

phagocytosis

10. The number of daughter cells formed when a cell undergoes mitosis is

_2_

11. The main energy compound of the cell is

_____

VIII. Practical Applications

Study each discussion. Then write the appropriate word or phrase in the space provided. The following are observations you might make while reviewing the work of a hospital laboratory.

1. The janitor in the laboratory was using a cleaning solution that contained ammonia. His activity caused ammonia molecules to spread throughout the room. The movement of molecules from an area of higher concentration to an area where their concentration is lower is called

diffusion

2. One of the laboratory technicians was trying to separate solid particles from a liquid mixture. He poured the mixture into a paper-lined funnel. The liquid flowed through the funnel while the solids remained behind on the paper. This process is called

_____

3. A laboratory technician was preparing to remove a tissue sample from a transport bottle containing normal saline. Normal saline was used for this purpose for the same reason that it is used in intravenous fluids, that is, it has the same concentration as the fluids in body cells. Such a solution is described as

isotonic

4. The laboratory technician was assisting in a community screening program for sickle cell disease. To perform this test, he examined slides containing a drop of blood with a reducing substance and another drop with normal saline. He suspected a mix-up in the test solutions because several slides had red cells that had ruptured. In scientific terms, the red cells had

Hypotonic

5. A patient was receiving concentrated fluid intravenously in the right arm. The nurse warned a phlebotomist drawing blood for laboratory tests to obtain the specimen from the left arm to avoid interference with test results. A solution that is more concentrated than body fluids is described as

Hypertonic

6. The genetic material in a blood sample was being examined for abnormality of the chromosomes. For these tests, the chromosomes are studied at the time of cell division. The name for this process of cell division is

mitosis

7. A sample of breast tissue was being examined to detect the presence of cancer cells. Breast cancer is an example of a disease that occurs more often within certain families than in others, suggesting that one cancer risk factor is

Hereditary

8. A young man was undergoing tests to determine the cause of his excessive thirst. The excess water he had consumed had passed through plasma membranes into many of his tissues. The process by which water passes through a semipermeable membrane is called

Plasma membrane

IX.   Short Essays

1. Name the two types of nucleic acids and briefly describe how they act in the cell.

DNA & RNA

2. Explain why the plasma membrane is described as selectively permeable.

3. Explain why it is important to keep cells in a solution that has the same concentration as the intracellular fluids.

_____

_____

_____

4. Explain what is meant by the term *risk factor* in cancer and list several of these factors.

_____

_____

_____

4

Tissues, Glands, and Membranes

I. Overview

The cell is the basic unit of life. Individual cells are grouped according to function into *tissues*. The four main groups of tissues include *epithelial tissue,* which forms glands, covers surfaces, and lines cavities; *connective tissue,* which gives structure and holds all parts of the body in place; *muscle tissue,* which produces movement; and *nervous tissue,* which conducts nerve impulses.

The simplest combination of tissues is a *membrane.* Membranes serve several purposes, a few of which are mentioned here: they may serve as dividing partitions, may line hollow organs and cavities, and may anchor various organs. Membranes that have epithelial cells on the surface are referred to as *epithelial membranes.* Two types of epithelial membranes are serous membranes, which line body cavities and cover the internal organs, and mucous membranes, which line passageways leading to the outside.

Connective tissue membranes cover or enclose organs, providing protection and support. These membranes include the fascia around muscles, the meninges around the brain and spinal cord and the tissues around the heart, bones, and cartilage.

Glands produce substances used by other cells and tissues. *Exocrine glands* produce secretions that are released through ducts to nearby parts of the body. *Endocrine glands* produce *hormones* that are carried by the blood to all parts of the body.

If the normal pattern of cell growth is disrupted by the formation of cells that multiply out of control, the result is a *tumor.* A tumor that is confined locally and does not spread is called a benign tumor; a tumor that spreads from its original site to other parts of the body, a process termed *metastasis,* is called a malignant tumor. Most benign tumors can be removed surgically; malignant tumors are usually treated by surgery, radiation, or chemotherapy, or by a combination of these methods.

II. Topics for Review

A. Classification of tissue
B. Functions of the four main types of tissues
C. Types of glands
D. Membranes
    1. Epithelial
    2. Connective tissue
E. Tumors
    1. Detection and treatment of cancer

III. Matching Exercises

Matching only within each group, write the answers in the spaces provided.

Group A

cilia	tissue	bone
adipose	exocrine	squamous
cartilage	stratified	

1. Term for glands that secrete through ducts   _____

2. A group of cells similar in structure and function   _____

3. Term that describes flat, irregular epithelial cells

_____

4. Tiny, hairlike projections from epithelium that can move dust and other foreign particles along the airways

_____

5. A type of connective tissue that stores fat and serves as a heat insulator

_____

6. A term that means *in layers*

_____

7. Tissue that forms when cartilage gradually becomes impregnated with calcium salts

_____

8. The hard connective tissue that acts as a shock absorber and as a bearing surface to reduce friction between moving parts

_____

Group B

ligament	collagen	neuron
fascia	transitional	mucus
cartilage		

1. The secretion that traps dust and other inhaled foreign particles

_____

2. A band or sheet of fibrous connective tissue around muscles

_____

3. The scientific name for a nerve cell

_____

4. The tough, elastic substance found at the ends of long bones

_____

5. Term for a wrinkled type of epithelium that is capable of great expansion

_____

6. The flexible white protein that makes up the main fibers in connective tissue

_____

7. A strong band of connective tissue that supports a joint

_____

Group C

myocardium	neurilemma	myelin
voluntary muscle	keloid	smooth muscle

1. The thin coating membrane that allows certain nerves to repair themselves

_____

2. The fatty insulating material that covers and protects some nerve fibers

_____

3. The thick, muscular layer of the heart wall

_____

4. The result of excess production of collagen in the formation of a scar

_____

5. Muscle tissue that forms the walls of the organs within the ventral body cavities

_____

6. Term used to describe skeletal muscle because it is usually under conscious control

_____

Group D

tendon	malignant	epithelium
suture	periosteum	benign
membrane	tumor	

1. Any thin sheet of tissue that separates two or more structures

_____

2. A layer of fibrous connective tissue around a bone

_____

3. The tissue that forms a protective covering for the body and that lines the digestive, respiratory, and urinary passages

_____

4. An abnormal tissue growth that may be caused by repeated injury to a single area

_____

5. A cord of connective tissue that connects a muscle to a bone

_____

6. To bring the edges of a wound together to aid healing and reduce the size of a scar

_____

7. Term that describes tumors that spread and grow rapidly, often causing death

_____

8. Term for a tumor that does not spread and is usually confined to a local area

_____

Group E

glands	pleura	mucous membranes
peritoneum	serous membranes	fascia
pericardium		

1. Types of membranes that line the closed cavities within the body

_____

2. The special sac that encloses the heart

_____

3. A tough membrane composed entirely of connective tissue that serves to anchor and support an organ or to cover a muscle

_____

4. The membrane that covers each lung

_____

5. The epithelial linings of tubes and spaces that are connected with the outside

_____

6. Specialized groups of cells that manufacture substances from blood components

_____

7. The large, serous membrane of the abdominal cavity

_____

Group F

synovial membrane	periosteum	superficial fascia
parietal layer	perichondrium	mucous membrane
mesothelium	capsule	cutaneous membrane

1. The tissue that underlies the skin

_____

2. The part of a serous membrane that is attached to the wall of a cavity or sac

_____

3. The lining of a joint cavity that produces secretions to reduce friction between the ends of bones

_____

4. The type of epithelium that covers serous membranes

_____

5. Another term for the skin

_____

6. The membrane that covers cartilage

_____

7. The type of lining found in the various parts of the respiratory tract

_____

8. The tough connective tissue membrane that covers a bone

_____

9. A tough, membranous connective tissue that encloses an organ

_____

Group G

sarcoma	lipoma	osteoma
carcinoma	myoma	glioma
nevus	angioma	

1. A benign connective tissue tumor that originates in adipose tissue

_____

2. The general term for a tumor composed of blood or lymphatic vessels

_____

3. A tumor that originates from the connective tissue of the central nervous system

_____

4. A benign connective tissue tumor that originates in a bone

_____

5. The scientific term for a mole or other small circumscribed tumor of the skin

_____

6. The most common type of cancer, one that originates in epithelium

_____

7. The type of cancer that originates in connective tissue and usually spreads by way of the bloodstream

_____

8. A tumor of muscle tissue that often appears as a fibroid in the uterus

_____

IV. Multiple Choice

Select the best answer and write the letter of your choice in the blank.

1. The study of tissues is

    a. microbiology
    b. endocrinology
    c. histology
    d. pharmacology
    e. cytology

1. _____

2. Which of the following is *not* a type of epithelial tissue?

    a. transitional
    b. squamous
    c. cuboidal
    d. columnar
    e. areolar

2. _____

3. The phrase *stratified squamous epithelium* describes

    a. flat, irregular, epithelial cells in a single layer
    b. square epithelial cells in many layers
    c. long, narrow, epithelial cells in a single layer
    d. simple, columnar, epithelial cells
    e. flat, irregular, epithelial cells in many layers

3. _____

4. Endocrine glands produce

    a. external secretions
    b. hormones
    c. digestive juices
    d. tears
    e. sweat

4. _____

5. A term that describes areolar connective tissue is

    a. loose
    b. keloid
    c. fascia
    d. adipose
    e. voluntary

5. _____

6. Adipose tissue stores

    a. mucus
    b. saliva
    c. cartilage
    d. fat
    e. bone

6. _____

7. The thin covering of some nerve fibers that aids in repair of a damaged nerve is the

    a. neuroglia
    b. neurilemma
    c. gray matter
    d. meninges
    e. fascia

7. _____

V. Labeling

For each of the following illustrations, write the name or names of each labeled part on the numbered lines.

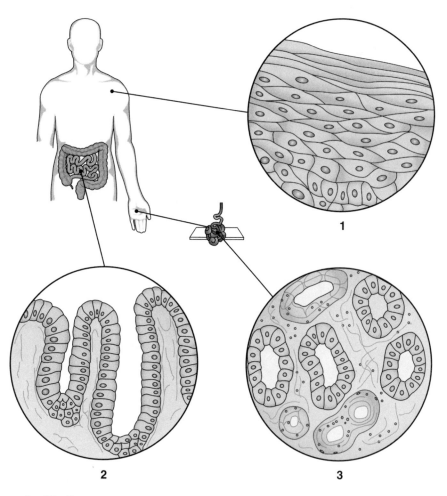

Three types of epithelium

1. _____   3. _____

2. _____

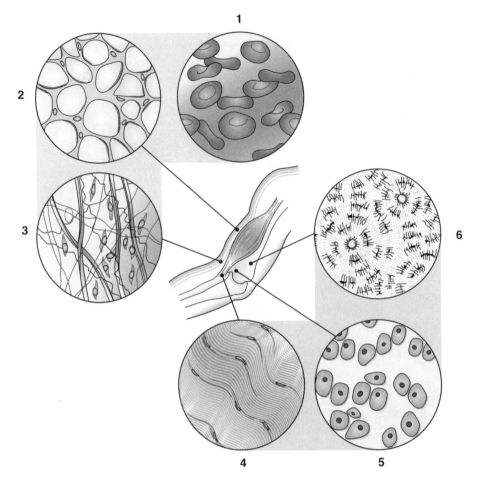

Connective tissue

1. _____   4. _____

2. _____   5. _____

3. _____   6. _____

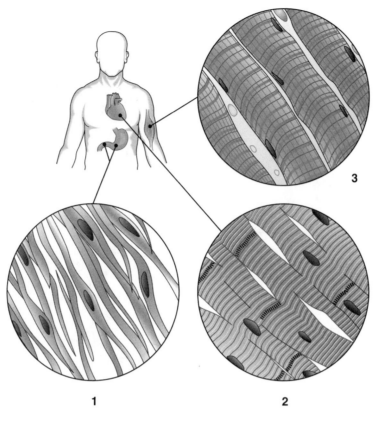

1

2

3

Muscle tissue

1. _____   3. _____

2. _____

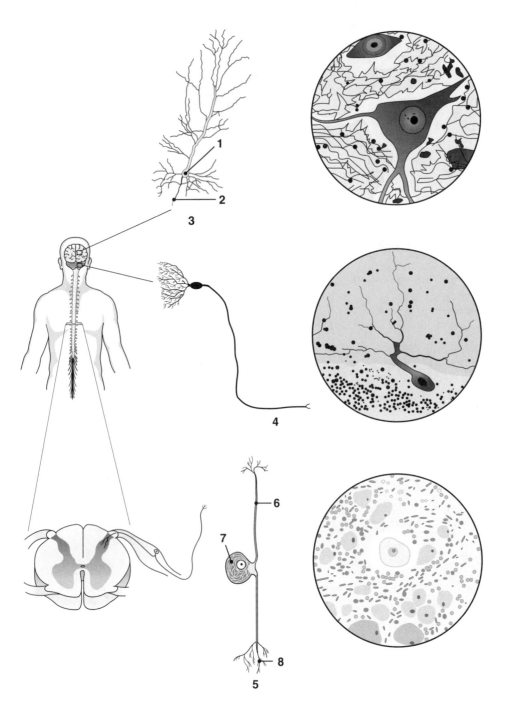

Nervous tissue

1. _____

2. _____

3. _____

4. _____

5. _____

6. _____

7. _____

8. _____

VI. True–False

For each question, write T for true or F for false in the blank to the left of each number. If a statement is false, correct it by replacing the underlined term and write the correct statement in the blanks below the question.

_____   1. Epithelium that is arranged in many layers is described as <u>simple</u>.

_____

_____

_____   2. <u>Smooth muscle</u> is also called visceral muscle.

_____

_____

_____   3. <u>Periosteum</u> is the membrane around a bone.

_____

_____

_____   4. A <u>tendon</u> connects a bone to another bone.

_____

_____

_____   5. The <u>endocrine glands</u> produce hormones.

_____

_____

_____   6. Sweat glands, tear glands, and sebaceous glands are all examples of <u>endocrine glands</u>.

_____

_____

_____   7. The <u>visceral</u> layer of a serous membrane lines the wall of a cavity or sac.

_____

_____

_____ 8. The <u>axon</u> of a neuron carries impulses toward the cell body.

_____

_____

_____ 9. A <u>carcinoma</u> is cancer of epithelial tissue.

_____

_____

VII. Completion Exercise

Write the word or phrase that correctly completes each sentence.

1. The basic unit of nervous tissue is the nerve cell, the
   scientific name for which is   _____

2. Movement is produced by the tissue known as   _____

3. The noun that means a serous membrane is   _____

4. Hormones enter the bloodstream and affect tissues distant
   from the glands that produce them. The glands that
   secrete hormones are known as the   _____

5. The supporting tissue of the body is called   _____

6. The only type of muscle that is voluntary is   _____

7. The lubricant produced by membranes that line cavities
   connected with the outside is called   _____

8. The tough connective tissue membrane that covers most
   parts of all bones is given the name   _____

9. A layer of tough, fibrous connective tissue that encloses
   an internal organ is called a(n)   _____

10. A lubricant that reduces friction between the ends of
    bones is produced by the   _____

11. The microscopic, hairlike projections found in the
    cells lining most of the respiratory tract are called   _____

12. The general term referring to a cancer that originates
    in epithelium and is spread through the lymphatic system is   _____

13. A malignant tumor that originates in connective tissue
    and that spreads by way of the bloodstream is called a(n)   _____

14. Among the forms of treatment of certain cancers is the
    use of drugs. This treatment is known as _____

VIII. Practical Applications

Study each discussion. Then write the appropriate word or phrase in the
space provided.

Group A

While observing in an outpatient clinic, a student noted the following cases.

1. Baby J experienced difficulty in breathing and had a copious
   discharge from his nose. A diagnosis of upper respiratory
   infection (URI) was made. The location of the membrane
   and the type of discharge indicated that the involved
   membrane was of a type known as a(n) _____

2. Mrs. K had suffered a crushing injury to the lower leg. Initially,
   she had little pain. Now, she complains of numbness and pain
   in the foot and leg. This type of injury is made worse by the
   tight, fibrous covering of the muscles, known as the _____

3. Mr. B was concerned about swelling and tenderness
   over his neck and upper back. His work involved the
   demolition of old buildings; he had become careless
   about personal cleanliness. Infection now involved
   the skin and connective tissue under it. The sheet
   of tissue that underlies the skin is called _____

4. Mrs. J had suffered a painful bump on her ankle. The
   swelling involved the superficial tissues and the
   fibrous covering of the bone, or the _____

5. Mrs. C had undergone surgery because of deformities
   due to rheumatoid arthritis, an inflammatory disorder
   of the membranes lining the joint spaces. The
   membrane lining a joint cavity is known as the _____

6. Ms. G experienced abdominal pains following longstanding
   infection of the pelvic organs. Connective tissue bands
   (adhesions) were found to extend throughout the
   peritoneal surface. The layer of peritoneum that is
   attached to the organs is called the _____

7. Student N suffered a mild concussion while playing football,
   and it was feared that there might be damage to the brain
   coverings. These brain and spinal cord coverings are known as _____

8. Mrs. J was quite ill. Her symptoms were those associated
   with the disease called lupus erythematosus. She complained
   that it hurt to breathe because the membranes covering
   the lungs were involved. The membrane covering each
   lung is the _____

Group B

A day in the tumor clinic involves observation of several patients. Among the situations you might encounter are the following.

1. Mr. B was concerned about a small skin growth on the left side of his face, which had not cleared after many months. He thought it might be growing. The physician informed Mr. B that a biopsy was necessary to make a positive diagnosis. If the growth proved to be a malignant epithelial tumor, it would be classified as a(n) _____

2. Mrs. C complained of an irritation in the area of a large dark mole on her right ankle. The physician advised her to have the mole removed and examined under the microscope, because such a mole may be malignant. This type of cancer is called a(n) _____

3. Mr. K's problem involved multiple, rounded growths located just under the skin of his right forearm. These were diagnosed as benign fatty tumors, or _____

4. Baby K was under treatment for a large birthmark on his right cheek. This type of tumor, which is composed of blood or lymphatic vessels, is classified as a(n) _____

5. Chad H was in clinic to receive a periodic chemotherapy for lymphoma. Lymphoma is a malignant neoplasm of _____

6. Mr. A's prostate cancer had been well controlled in the previous year with radiation therapy. He was in the clinic on this day for a follow-up PSA test. This is one of several tests for products produced in excess by tumors. Such tests are done for diagnosis or to monitor treated patients for return of disease. The specimen in which these products are measured is the _____

IX. Short Essays

1. Define *epithelial tissue*. Describe the different types of epithelial tissue and give several examples.

    _____

    _____

    _____

2. Compare exocrine and endocrine glands and give examples of each type.

_____

_____

_____

3. Define *connective tissue,* and describe its role in the body, citing several examples of connective tissue.

_____

_____

_____

4. Compare epithelial and connective tissue membranes and give several examples of each.

_____

_____

_____

Unit II

DISEASE AND THE FIRST LINE OF DEFENSE

5

Disease and Disease-Producing Organisms

I. Overview

Disease may be defined as an abnormality of the structure or function of a part, organ, or system. The categories of disease are many and varied. Among them are infections, degenerative diseases, nutritional disorders, metabolic disorders, immune disorders, neoplasms, and psychiatric disorders. Predisposing causes are factors that play a part in the development of disease, such as age, sex, heredity, environmental factors, and emotional disturbance. An understanding of disease incorporates a study of the body including its anatomy (structure) and its physiology (functions) under normal and pathologic (abnormal) conditions. This understanding is aided by use of disease terminology.

   Infection, or invasion of the body by disease-producing microorganisms, including bacteria, fungi, viruses, and protozoa, is the most important cause of disease in human beings. A second major cause of human disease is *infestation,* a type of infection due to parasitic worms. Control of infection depends on understanding how organisms are transmitted and how they enter and leave the body. Public health has been vastly improved through laboratory identification of pathogens and the application of *aseptic* and *chemotherapeutic* methods to prevent or control their spread.

II. Topics for Review

A. Categories of disease
B. Predisposing causes of disease
C. Disease terminology
D. Steps in treatment
E. Microorganisms
F. Parasitic worms

G. Microbial control
   1. Chemotherapy
   2. Laboratory identification of pathogens

III. Matching Exercises

Matching only within each group, write the answers in the spaces provided.

Group A

systemic	chronic	therapy
symptom	acute	sign
pathogen	helminth	

1. A disease-causing organism   _____

2. Describing a relatively severe disorder of short duration   _____

3. A condition of disease that is experienced by the patient   _____

4. A course of treatment   _____

5. Term for a disease that persists over a long period   _____

6. Scientific name for a worm   _____

7. Evidence of disease that can be observed by others   _____

8. Term for a generalized infection   _____

Group B

cocci   ascaris   curved rods
fungi   rickettsias   viruses
protozoa   bacilli   chlamydias

1. Spherical bacteria   _____

2. Group of bacteria that includes the cholera organism   _____

3. Group of small bacteria that includes the agents causing trachoma and parrot fever   _____

4. Group of organisms that includes yeasts and molds   _____

5. Rod-shaped bacteria   _____

6. The group of microorganisms described as animal-like   _____

7. Group of parasites that includes the agents causing typhus fever and Rocky Mountain spotted fever   _____

8. The smallest known infectious agents   _____

9. A large roundworm   _____

Group C

etiology   incidence   idiopathic
diagnosis   epidemic   endemic
asepsis   sterilization   syndrome

1. The process that kills every living organism on an object   _____

2. The process of determining the nature of an illness   _____

3. A group of signs or symptoms that occur together   _____

4. Term for a disease present at the same time in many people living in the same area   _____

5. Term for a disorder without known cause, or self-originating   _____

6. The study of the cause of a disorder   _____

7. The range of occurrence of a disease and its tendency to affect particular groups of people   _____

8. Term for a disease that is present continuously in a given area   _____

9. A condition in which no disease-causing organisms are present   _____

Group D

prognosis   opportunistic   parasitology
microbiology   communicable   physiology
pathology   protozoology   bacteriology

1. The study of organisms that live on or within other organisms at the expense of those organisms   _____

2. The study that deals with the activities or functions of a living organism   _____

3. The study of all microscopic organisms   _____

4. The field that includes study of rickettsias and chlamydias   _____

5. Term for an infection that takes hold in a weakened host   _____

6. The study that deals with the nature of disease and includes the changes caused by disease   _____

7. Term for a disease that can be transmitted from one person to another   _____

8. A prediction of the probable outcome of a disease   _____

9. The study of one-celled animals   _____

Group E

infestation   spore   pasteurization
pandemic   infection   antibiotic
tuberculosis   chemotherapy   botulism

1. Invasion of the body by pathogenic microorganisms   _____

2. A deadly type of food poisoning due to a rod-shaped bacillus   _____

3. The process of heating milk to 145°F for 30 minutes and then allowing it to cool rapidly before it is packaged   _____

4. Invasion by a parasitic worm   _____

5. A disease caused by an acid-fast organism   _____

6. Treatment of a disease by the administration of a chemical agent   _____

7. A resistant form of bacterium   _____

8. A disease that is prevalent over a very large area of the world   _____

9. A chemical agent derived from living cells that is used to kill or arrest the growth of pathogens   _____

IV. Multiple Choice

Select the best answer and write the letter of your choice in the blank.

1. Cancers and other types of tumors are termed   1. _____

   a. congenital
   b. preexisting
   c. neoplasms
   d. therapeutic
   e. acid-fast

2. Blood poisoning is a generalized infection described as   2. _____

   a. aseptic
   b. benign
   c. nosocomial
   d. local
   e. systemic

3. Which of the following sciences is *not* included in the science of microbiology?   3. _____

   a. mycology
   b. virology
   c. helminthology
   d. bacteriology
   e. protozoology

4. The sexually transmitted disease gonorrhea is caused by round bacteria that occur in pairs. These are   4. _____

   a. streptococci
   b. bacilli
   c. spirochetes
   d. diplococci
   e. staphylococci

5. Athlete's foot, tinea capitis, thrush, and *Candida* infections are all caused by   5. _____

   a. viruses
   b. fungi
   c. rickettsias
   d. worms
   e. filariae

6. Which of the following is true of an anaerobic organism?   6. _____

   a. It is airborne.
   b. It requires oxygen for growth.
   c. It cannot produce toxins.
   d. It can grow in the absence of oxygen.
   e. It is not pathogenic.

7. The normal flora consists of organisms that

    a. normally grow on or in the body
    b. cause infections
    c. are resistant to antibiotics
    d. produce antibiotics
    e. have a short life span

7. _____

8. Pinworms, hookworms, trichina, and filaria are examples of

    a. flatworms
    b. flagellates
    c. flukes
    d. roundworms
    e. ciliates

8. _____

9. An autoclave is a device that is used to

    a. pasteurize milk
    b. disinfect surfaces
    c. achieve bacteriostasis
    d. treat an opportunistic infection
    e. sterilize equipment

9. _____

V. Labeling

For each of the following illustrations, write the name or names of each labeled part on the numbered lines.

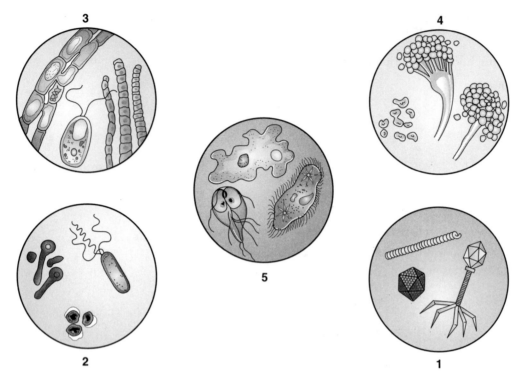

Examples of microorganisms

1. _____   4. _____

2. _____   5. _____

3. _____

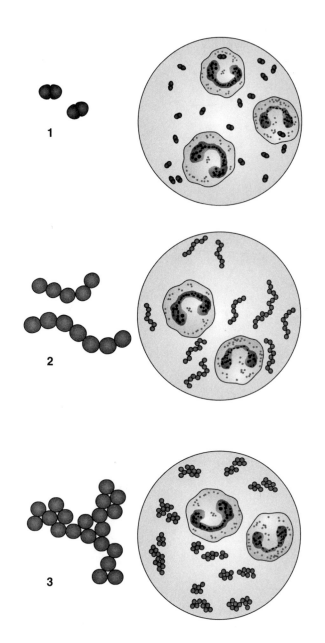

Spherical bacteria

1. _____   3. _____

2. _____

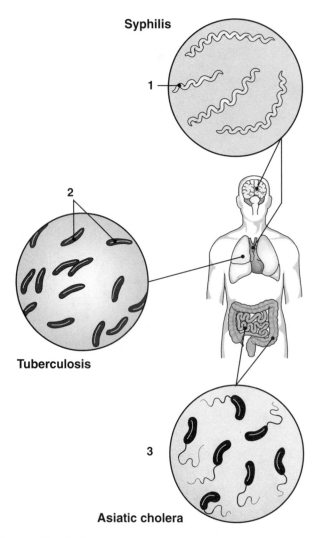

Syphilis

1

2

Tuberculosis

3

Asiatic cholera

Rod-shaped and curved bacteria

1. _____   3. _____

2. _____

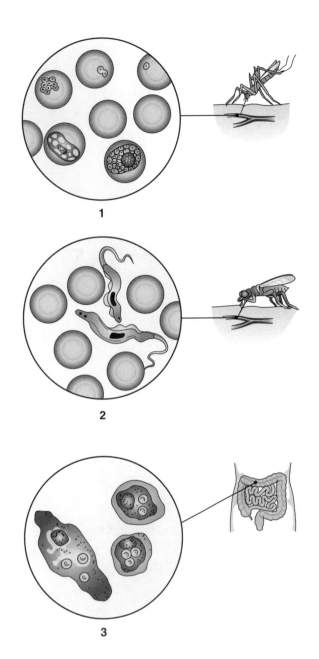

Pathogenic protozoa

1. _____   3. _____

2. _____

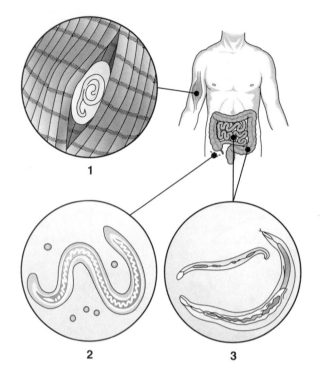

1. _____

2. _____

3. _____

Common parasitic worms

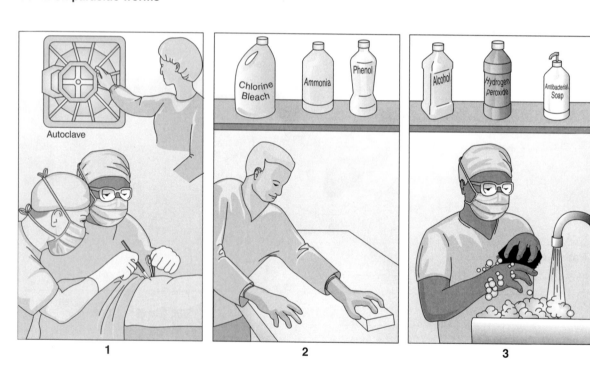

Aseptic methods

1. _____   3. _____

2. _____

VI. True–False

For each question, write T for true or F for false in the blank to the left of each number. If a statement is false, correct it by replacing the underlined term and write the correct statement in the blanks below the question.

_____ 1. An <u>acute</u> disease is one that continues or recurs for long periods.

_____

_____

_____ 2. Mycology is the study of <u>fungi</u>.

_____

_____

_____ 3. An <u>anaerobic</u> organism requires oxygen for growth.

_____

_____

_____ 4. An acid-fast organism <u>retains</u> color (stain) after application of an acid.

_____

_____

_____ 5. Gram-<u>positive</u> organisms appear bluish purple under the microscope.

_____

_____

_____ 6. <u>Disinfection</u> kills every living organism on or in an object.

_____

_____

VII. Completion Exercise

Write the word or phrase that correctly completes each sentence.

1. An insect or other animal that transmits a disease-causing organism from one host to another is a(n) _____

2. Pneumonia, meningitis, and rheumatic fever are caused by round bacteria known as _____

3. Legionnaire's disease, tuberculosis, and tetanus (lockjaw) are caused by rod-shaped microorganisms known as

_____

4. Chickenpox, hepatitis, the common cold, and many other contagious diseases are caused by submicroscopic organisms known as

_____

5. Tetanus is caused by an organism that exists in two forms. One of these is the growing vegetative form. The other is a resting and resistant form, the

_____

6. Asiatic cholera is a disease found in India, China, and other Asiatic countries. It is caused by a comma-shaped microorganism called

_____

7. Syphilis is a sexually transmitted disease that may eventually involve the brain and circulatory organs. It is caused by a corkscrew-shaped microorganism called a(n)

_____

8. Bacteria that are pathogenic may cause injury and even death by the action of poisons referred to as

_____

9. Included in the class of protozoa called *Sporozoa* is a plasmodium that causes a debilitating tropical disease called

_____

10. A small roundworm that may become enclosed in a cyst or sac inside the muscles of the pig and be transmitted to humans by way of improperly cooked pork causes a disease called

_____

11. The flatworm composed of many segments (proglottids) may grow to a length of 50 feet—hence the name

_____

VIII. Practical Applications

Study each discussion. Then write the appropriate word or phrase in the space provided.

1. Ms. C's case required further study. She had an obscure disorder for which no cause had been found. Such a disease is often referred to as

_____

2. Mr. S needed prophylactic (preventive) treatment because he had received several puncture wounds while repairing an old building. He was given an injection to prevent the development of lockjaw. The scientific name for lockjaw is

_____

3. Young Ashley was brought to the clinic with complaints of sore throat, fever, and earache. The health care practitioner took a throat swab and returned in 10 minutes with the result. The sore throat was due to a common organism from a group of chain-forming spherical bacteria known as

_____

72

4. The health care practitioner tested to ensure that the sore throat (acute pharyngitis) was due to a type of bacterium susceptible to antibiotics. This precaution in the ordering of antibiotics helps reduce the development of strains of microorganisms that do not respond to antibiotics and are described as _____

5. Mrs. A brought her young daughter to the clinic for examination of boils (furuncles) that had been appearing on the child's neck with disturbing frequency. Boils are often due to round microorganisms that resemble bunches of grapes when examined under the microscope. These organisms are called _____

6. Mr. E came to the clinic because he had suffered from bouts of diarrhea since returning from a camping trip that took him into several countries. One common cause of intestinal disorder is an amoeba (*Entamoeba histolytica*) that produces a disease called _____

7. Mrs. K had a fever, cough, and other symptoms of pneumonia. The suspected portal of entry for the organisms causing her illness is the _____

8. Mr. L came to the clinic for administration of drugs used to treat his condition of Hodgkin's disease, a type of cancer. Drugs used in treatment of cancer are known as _____

IX. Short Essays

1. Define the term *predisposing cause* in relation to disease, and give several examples of predisposing causes.

   _____

   _____

   _____

2. What is the science of pathophysiology, and why is it important in medicine?

   _____

   _____

   _____

3. Describe some disadvantages of drug therapy.

   _____

   _____

   _____

6

The Skin in Health and Disease

I. Overview

Because of its various properties, the skin can be classified as a membrane, an organ, or a system. The outermost layer of the skin is the *epidermis*. Beneath the epidermis is the *dermis* (the true skin) where the skin glands and other appendages are mainly located. The *subcutaneous tissue* underlies the skin. It contains fat that serves as insulation. The appendages of the skin are the *sudoriferous* (sweat) *glands*, the oil-secreting *sebaceous glands*, the hair, and nails.

The skin protects deeper tissues against drying and against invasion by harmful organisms. It regulates body temperature through evaporation of sweat and loss of heat at the surface. It collects information from the environment by means of sensory receptors.

The protein *keratin* in the epidermis thickens and protects the skin and makes up hair and nails. *Melanin* is the main pigment that gives the skin its color. It functions to filter out harmful ultraviolet radiation from the sun. The color of the skin is also influenced by such factors as the quantity of blood circulating in the surface blood vessels and its hemoglobin concentration.

Much can be learned about the condition of the skin by observing for discoloration, injury, or lesions. Aging, exposure to sunlight, and the health of other body systems also have a bearing on the condition and appearance of the skin. The skin is subject to numerous diseases, common forms of which are atopic dermatitis (eczema), acne, infections, and cancer.

II. Topics for Review

A. Skin layers
   1. Epidermis

        2. Dermis
            a. Subcutaneous layer
B. Skin glands
    1. Sudoriferous glands
    2. Sebaceous glands
C. Hair and nails
D. Functions of the skin
E. Observation of the skin
F. Skin diseases

III.   Matching Exercises

Matching only within each group, write the answers in the spaces provided.

Group A

melanin   sebaceous gland   integument
epidermis   sudoriferous gland   keratin
ciliary gland   dermis

1. Another name for the skin as a whole   <u>integument</u>

2. A gland that produces sweat   <u>sudoriferous</u>

3. A gland that produces an oily secretion on skin and hair   <u>sebaceous</u>

4. The protein in the epidermis that thickens and protects
   the skin   <u>keratin</u>

5. The outermost part of the skin, formed by several layers of epithelial cells — *epidermis*

6. The true skin, or corium — *dermis*

7. The pigment that is largely responsible for skin color — *melain*

8. A modified sweat gland found at the edge of the eyelid — *ciliary*

Group B

lesion   connective tissue   dermis
receptor   erythema   infection
subcutaneous tissue

1. Redness of the skin — *erythema*

2. The tissue that composes the framework of the dermis — *connective*

3. A sensory nerve ending in the skin that responds to information from the environment — *receptor*

4. The tissue layer under the true skin — *subcutaneous*

5. A wound or local damage to the skin — *lesion*

6. The layer of the skin that contains most of the glands and hair — *dermis*

7. A condition that may follow a wound or injury to the skin — *infection*

Group C

papillae   stratum corneum   wax
follicle   sebum   nerve endings
stratum germinativum   melanin

1. The uppermost layer of the epidermis —

2. Secretion of the ceruminous glands — *wax*

3. Portions of the dermis that extend into the epidermis — *papillae*

4. The pigment that increases when the skin is exposed to sunlight — *melanin*

5. The oily secretion of the sebaceous glands — *sebum*

6. The deepest layer of the epidermis, which contains living, dividing cells — *stratum germinativum*

7. Structures in the skin that obtain information about the environment — *nerve ending*

8. The sheath in which a hair develops — *follicle*

Group D

~~papule~~	vesicle	dermatitis
pruritus	macule	laceration
~~ulcer~~	urticaria	

1. Any inflammation of the skin _____

2. Any flat, discolored spot on the skin _____macule_____

3. A sore associated with disintegration and death of tissue _____ulcer_____

4. A small sac that contains fluid; a blister _____

5. A firm, raised area of the skin, such as a pimple _____papule_____

6. Another term for itching _____

7. A rough, jagged tear in the skin _____laceration_____

8. An allergic disorder associated with red, raised, itchy patches (hives) _____

IV. Multiple Choice

Select the best answer and write the letter of your choice in the blank.

1. The subcutaneous layer of the skin is composed mainly of fibrous connective tissue and

   a. nervous tissue
   b. cartilage
   c. epithelial tissue
   d. adipose tissue
   e. muscle tissue

   1. _____a_____

2. A yellowish discoloration that may be due to the presence of bile pigments in the blood is called

   a. eczema
   b. melanin
   c. impetigo
   d. alopecia
   e. jaundice

   2. _____e_____

3. Which of the following is *not* a function of skin?

   a. protection
   b. breathing
   c. prevention of drying
   d. temperature regulation
   e. detection of changes in the environment

   3. _____b_____

4. When blood vessels enlarge, they are said to

    a. dilate
    b. constrict
    c. become narrower
    d. close
    e. merge

4. _____a_____

5. A discoloration of the skin caused by diet is

    a. pallor
    b. cyanosis
    c. liver spots
    d. carotenemia
    e. dermatosis

5. _____d_____

6. The term *bedsore* is the common name for a

    a. laceration
    b. macule
    c. decubitus ulcer
    d. psoriasis
    e. herpes

6. _____c_____

7. A modified sweat gland that produces ear wax is the

    a. ciliary gland
    b. ceruminous gland
    c. sudoriferous gland
    d. corneal gland
    e. stasis gland

7. _____b_____

V. Labeling

For each of the following illustrations, write the name or names of each labeled part on the numbered lines.

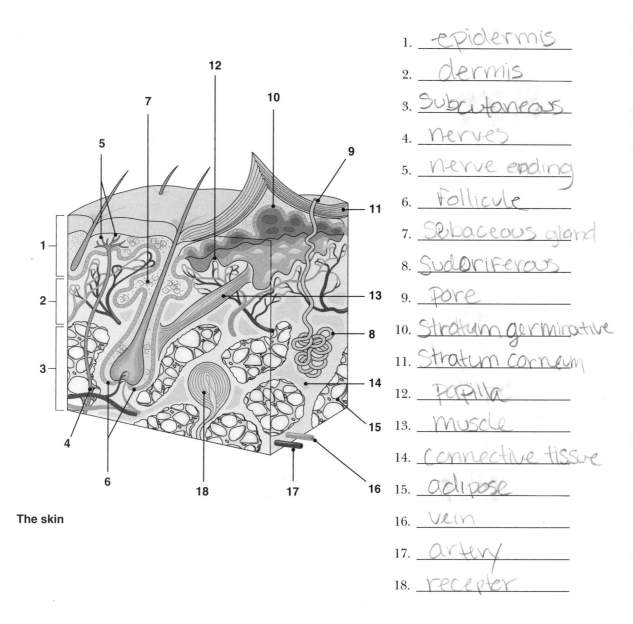

The skin

1. epidermis
2. dermis
3. Subcutaneous
4. nerves
5. nerve ending
6. follicle
7. sebaceous gland
8. Sudoriferous
9. pore
10. Stratum germinative
11. Stratum corneum
12. Papilla
13. muscle
14. connective tissue
15. adipose
16. vein
17. artery
18. recepter

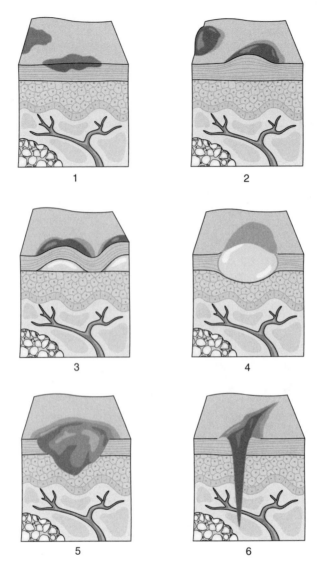

Some common skin lesions

1. macules

2. papules

3. vesicles

4. pustules

5. ulcer

6. laceration

VI. True–False

For each question, write T for true or F for false in the blank to the left of each number. If a statement is false, correct it by replacing the underlined term and write the correct statement in the blanks below the question.

F 1. The <u>stratum corneum</u> is the lowermost layer of the epidermis.

Stratum germinative

F 2. To conserve heat, the blood vessels in the skin <u>dilate</u>.

They constrict

T 3. The subcutaneous tissue is also called the <u>superficial fascia</u>.

T 4. Sebum is produced by <u>sudoriferous glands</u>.

T 5. <u>Keratin</u> is a protein that helps to thicken the skin.

VII. Completion Exercise

Write the word or phrase that correctly completes each sentence.

1. The outer layer of the epidermis, the cells of which are constantly being shed, is designated the horny layer, or _____

2. Many kinds of irritants and pathogens cause skin inflammation. The general term for this disorder is _dermatitis_

3. The main pigment of the skin is _melanin_

4. Epidermophytosis, or athlete's foot, is due to infection by _fungi_

5. Numerous factors including infection may cause baldness. Absence of hair from any areas where it is normally present is called _alopecia_

6. An acute contagious skin disease caused by staphylococci or streptococci may be extremely serious in infants and young children. This disease is _____

7. Overactivity of the sebaceous glands during adolescence may play a part in the common skin disease called _____

8. The general term for a diffuse area of redness of the skin is _____

9. The ceruminous glands and the ciliary glands are modified forms of _____

10. Hair and nails are composed mainly of a protein named _keratin_

11. The blood vessels that nourish the epidermis are located in the skin layer just below the epidermis. This deeper layer is called the _____

VIII. Practical Applications

Study each discussion. Then write the appropriate word or phrase in the space provided.

Group A

These patients were seen in the outpatient clinic.

1. Mrs. A brought her three children to the clinic. The 9-month-old baby had redness of both cheeks, a symptom that the physician described as _____

2. The physician also found several tiny blisters on the baby's cheeks. Her notation on the chart referred to these eruptions as _____

3. On both of the baby's cheeks, there were small, pimple-like protrusions. The physician referred to them as _____

4. The physician diagnosed a common noncontagious disorder of sensitive skin known as _____

5. Mrs. A's 6-year-old son had a number of blisters on his hands that contained pus. Microscopic examination revealed the presence of staphylococci. This contagious skin disease is called _____

6. Mrs. A wondered why her own skin looked more yellow than normal. Questioning revealed that she had become a food faddist and was eating carrots and other deeply colored vegetables to the exclusion of other foods. Mrs. A's condition is called _____

7. L, age 15, came to the clinic with his father. The boy's skin was marked by pimples and blackheads and had a roughened appearance. This common disorder of the oil glands is found mainly in adolescents and is called

_____

Group B

1. Mr. K, age 38, was losing his hair. He mentioned that many of his male relatives had a similar problem. The medical term for baldness is

_____

2. Numerous vesicles and ulcers were found on Mrs. D's feet. This disorder is popularly called *athlete's foot.* The medical term for it is

_____

3. Mrs. J was concerned about a redness and silvery scaling on her elbows that seemed to ''come and go.'' The name for this disorder is

_____

4. Mr. M, a laborer, had neglected to give his skin proper care. Numerous painful nodules were seen in the axillae (armpits). These nodules, due to bacteria entering the hair follicles, are called boils, or

_____

5. There was also a deep-seated, draining infection of the subcutaneous tissue on Mr. M's lower back. This type of pus-producing lesion is known as a(n)

_____

6. Fair-skinned Mr. G had spent most of his 40 years in Arizona and southeastern California. He now noticed a firm nodule on the edge of the left ear and said it was increasing in size. Biopsy revealed a common form of cancer known as basal cell

_____

7. Mr. G's teenage son had large areas of red, peeling skin due to sunburn. The nurse advised use of sunscreen to prevent damage and premature aging of the skin, as well as cancer of pigment-forming cells, a type of malignancy called

_____

IX. Short Essays

1. Explain why the skin is valuable in diagnosis.

_____

_____

_____

2. Name several pigments that can give color to skin, and identify their sources.

_____

_____

_____

3. Describe the changes that may occur in skin with aging.

_____

_____

_____

Unit III

MOVEMENT AND SUPPORT

7

The Skeleton: Bones and Joints

I. Overview

The skeletal system protects and supports the body parts and serves as an attachment for the muscles, which furnish the power for movement. The bones also store calcium salts and are the site of blood cell production. The skeletal system includes some 206 bones; the number varies slightly according to age and the individual.

Although bone tissue contains a matrix of nonliving material, bones also contain living cells and have their own systems of blood vessels, lymphatic vessels, and nerves. Bone tissue may be either *spongy* or *compact*. Compact bone is found in the shaft (diaphysis) of a long bone and in the outer layer of other bones. Spongy bone makes up the ends (epiphyses) of a long bone and the center of other bones. *Red marrow,* present at the ends of long bones and the center of other bones, manufactures blood cells; *yellow marrow,* which is largely fat, is found in the central cavities of the long bones.

Bone tissue is produced by cells called *osteoblasts,* which gradually convert cartilage to bone during development. The mature cells that maintain bone are called *osteocytes,* and the cells that break down bone for remodeling and repair are the *osteoclasts.*

The skeleton is divided into two main groups of bones, the *axial skeleton* and the *appendicular skeleton.* The axial skeleton includes the skull, spinal column, ribs, and sternum. The appendicular skeleton consists of the bones of the arms and legs, the shoulder girdle, and the pelvic girdle. Disorders of bones include metabolic disorders, tumors, infection, structural disorders, and fractures.

A *joint* is the region of union of two or more bones; joints are classified according to structure and to the degree of movement permitted. *Synovial joints* show the greatest degree of movement. The six types of synovial joints allow for a variety of movements in different directions. Connective tissue bands, *ligaments,* hold the bones together in all the synovial joints and many of the less movable joints.

II. Topics for Review

A. Functions of bones
B. Structure of bone
    1. Bone cells
C. Bone growth and repair
D. Bone markings
E. Bones of the axial skeleton
F. Bones of the appendicular skeleton
G. Disorders of bones
H. Types of joints
    1. Movements at synovial joints
I. Disorders of joints

III. Matching Exercises

Matching only within each group, write the answers in the spaces provided.

Group A

osteoblast	red marrow	appendicular skeleton
periosteum	cartilage	endosteum
axial skeleton	yellow marrow	

1. The thin membrane that lines the central cavity of long bones _____ *~~yellow~~ red marrow*

2. The fatty material found inside the central cavities of long bones _____ *yellow marrow*

3. The bony framework of the head and trunk together _____

4. A cell that produces bone _____ *osteoblast*

5. The material that forms most of the embryonic skeleton _____

6. The group of bones that forms the framework for the extremities, shoulder, and hip _____ *Axial skeleton*

7. The tough connective tissue membrane that covers bones _____ *Periosteum*

8. The site of blood cell production _____

Group B

parietal bone   temporal bone   frontal bone
sphenoid bone   occipital bone   ethmoid bone

1. The bat-shaped bone that extends behind the eyes and also forms part of the base of the skull _____

2. The bone that forms the lower side and part of the base of the central area of the skull _____

3. The bone that forms the forehead _____

4. The bone located between the eyes that extends into the nasal cavity, eye sockets, and cranial floor _____

5. The bone that forms the larger part of the upper and side walls of the cranium _____

6. The bone that forms the back of the skull and part of the base of the skull _____

Group C

zygomatic bone   maxilla   mandible
hyoid   nasal bone   lacrimal bone

1. The bone that forms the upper part of the cheek _____

2. The very small bone at the inside corner of the eye _____

3. The U-shaped bone lying just below the skull proper _____

4. The only movable bone of the skull _____

5. A slender bone that forms the bridge of the nose _____

6. A bone of the upper jaw _____

Group D

collagen   cervical region   thoracic region
lumbar region   coccyx   scoliosis
diaphysis   floating ribs   true ribs

1. The second part of the vertebral column, made up of 12 vertebrae

    _____

2. The shaft of a long bone

    _____

3. The tail part of the vertebral column, made of four or five small fused bones

    _____

4. The fibrous protein that gives strength and resilience to bone tissue

    _____

5. A lateral curvature of the vertebral column

    _____

6. The third section of the vertebral column, consisting of five large vertebrae

    _____

7. Term for the first seven pairs of ribs as a group

    _____

8. The region of the spinal cord made up of the first seven vertebrae and comprising the main framework of the neck

    _____

9. The last two pairs of false ribs, which are very short and do not extend to the front of the body

    _____

Group E

kyphosis   foramina   lordosis
matrix   sacrum   fontanel
spongy bone   costal

1. An adjective that refers to the ribs

    _____

2. Openings or holes that extend into or through bones

    _____

3. The type of bone tissue found at the ends of a long bone

    _____

4. A soft spot in the infant skull that later closes

    _____

5. The material between the cells in bone tissue

    _____

6. The region of the spinal column below the lumbar region, composed of four to five fused bones

    _____

7. An abnormally increased concave curvature of the thoracic spine

    _____

8. An excessive anterior convexity of the lumbar curve

    _____

Group F

patella   epiphysis   olecranon
ulna   tibia   radius
fibula

1. The lateral bone of the leg   _____

2. The end of a long bone   _____

3. The medial forearm bone   _____

4. The upper part of the ulna, which forms the point of the elbow   _____

5. The scientific name for the kneecap   _____

6. The bone located on the thumb side of the forearm   _____

7. The larger of the two leg bones   _____

Group G

ligament   greater trochanter   carpal bones
metacarpal bones   calcaneus   ilium
clavicle   phalanges

1. The upper wing-shaped part of the os coxae in the pelvic girdle   _____

2. A bone of the shoulder girdle   _____

3. The five bones in the palm of the hand   _____

4. The largest of the tarsal bones; the heel bone   _____

5. A connective tissue band that holds bones together at a joint   _____

6. The bones of the wrist   _____

7. The 14 small bones that form the framework of the fingers on each hand   _____

8. The large, rounded projection at the upper and lateral portion of the femur   _____

Group H

impacted fracture   osteitis deformans   comminuted fracture
greenstick fracture   spiral fracture   open fracture
osteomyelitis   bursitis

1. Another name for Paget's disease, a disorder that involves an abnormality of calcium metabolism   _____

2. An infection of bone caused by pus-producing bacteria   _____

3. An incomplete break in a bone that is most likely to occur in children

    _____

4. A fracture in which the broken ends of the bones are jammed into each other

    _____

5. A fracture in which a wound penetrates to a broken bone or a broken bone protrudes through the skin

    _____

6. Inflammation of a small sac near a joint

    _____

7. A fracture in which a bone has been twisted apart

    _____

8. A break in which there is more than one fracture line and bone is splintered or crushed

    _____

Group I

articular cartilage	flexion	synovial
rotation	abduction	ball-and-socket
extension	hinge	

1. The reverse of flexion

    _____

2. Movement away from the midline of the body

    _____

3. Motion around a central axis

    _____

4. Term for the lubricating fluid inside a joint cavity

    _____

5. The type of joint that allows for circumduction

    _____

6. The type of joint found at the elbow

    _____

7. The protective layer of tissue that covers the contacting bone surfaces at a joint

    _____

8. A bending motion that decreases the angle between two parts

    _____

Group J

resorption	articulation	diarthrosis
ossification	rheumatoid arthritis	acetabulum
diaphysis	osteoporosis	

1. A common disorder in older women, which involves abnormal bone metabolism

    _____

2. The shaft of a long bone

    _____

3. The deep socket in the hip bone that holds the head of the femur

    _____

4. The breakdown of bone tissue

    _____

5. The region of union of two or more bones; a joint   _____

6. A crippling inflammatory disease of joints   _____

7. The process of bone formation   _____

8. A freely movable joint   _____

IV. Multiple Choice

Select the best answer and write the letter of your choice in the blank.

1. The hard bone matrix is composed mainly of salts of the element   1. _____

   a. iodine
   b. sodium
   c. calcium
   d. chlorine
   e. nitrogen

2. The part of the skull that encloses the brain is the   2. _____

   a. vomer
   b. hyoid bone
   c. sinus
   d. conchae
   e. cranium

3. A joint between bones of the skull is a   3. _____

   a. trochanter
   b. crest
   c. malleolus
   d. suture
   e. cleft

4. Which of the following is *not* a depression or hole in a bone?   4. _____

   a. process
   b. fossa
   c. foramen
   d. sinus
   e. meatus

5. The sella turcica, which holds the pituitary gland, is part of the   5. _____

   a. ethmoid
   b. maxilla
   c. sphenoid
   d. parietal
   e. hyoid

6. The patella is the largest of a type of bone that develops within a tendon or a joint capsule. It is described as

    a. sesamoid
    b. axial
    c. tarsal
    d. symphysis
    e. axial

6. _____

7. The spine, acromion, glenoid cavity, and coracoid process are part of the

    a. humerus
    b. sternum
    c. tibia
    d. scapula
    e. os coxae

7. _____

8. The lower end of the sternum, used as a landmark for cardiopulmonary resuscitation, is the

    a. ischial spine
    b. xiphoid process
    c. infraspinous fossa
    d. tarsus
    e. lateral malleolus

8. _____

9. The foramen magnum is

    a. a large hole in a hip bone near the symphysis pubis
    b. the curved rim along the top of the hip bone
    c. a hole between vertebrae that allows for passage of a spinal nerve
    d. a process on the temporal bone
    e. a large opening at the base of the skull through which the spinal cord passes

9. _____

10. Which is *not* an example of a synovial joint?

    a. condyloid
    b. pivot
    c. gliding
    d. saddle
    e. symphysis

10. _____

V. Labeling

For each of the following illustrations, write the name or names of each labeled part on the numbered lines.

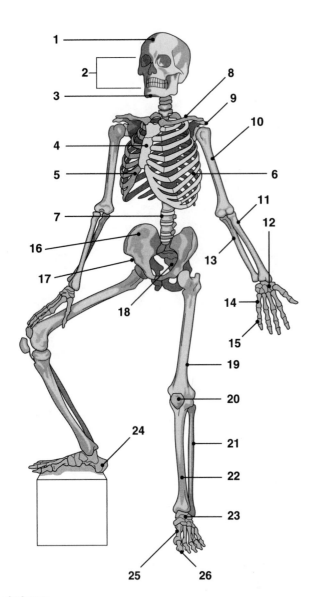

The skeleton

1. _____

2. _____

3. _____

4. _____

5. _____

6. _____

7. _____

8. _____

9. _____

10. _____

11. _____

12. _____

13. _____

14. _____

15. _____

16. _____

17. _____

18. _____

19. _____

20. _____

21. _____

22. _____

23. _____

24. _____

25. _____

26. _____

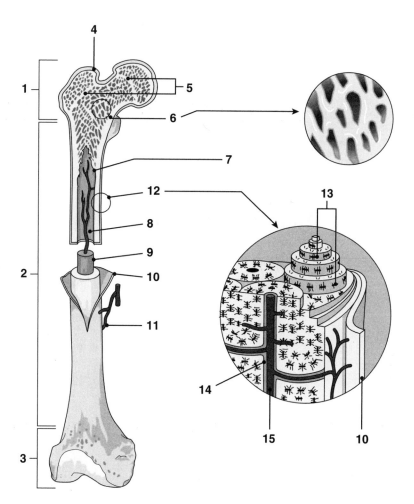

Structure of a long bone

1. _____

2. _____

3. _____

4. _____

5. _____

6. _____

7. _____

8. _____

9. _____

10. _____

11. _____

12. _____

13. _____

14. _____

15. _____

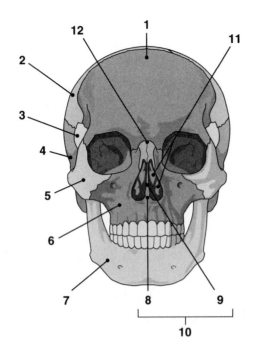

Skull from the front

1. _____

2. _____

3. _____

4. _____

5. _____

6. _____

7. _____

8. _____

9. _____

10. _____

11. _____

12. _____

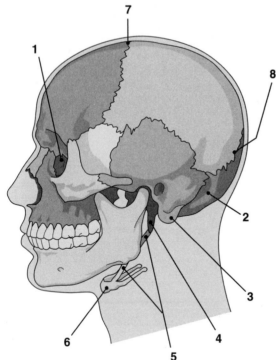

Skull from the left

1. _____

2. _____

3. _____

4. _____

5. _____

6. _____

7. _____

8. _____

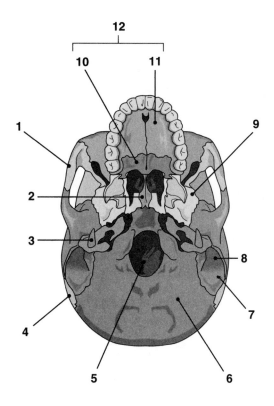

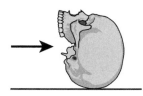

Skull from below, lower jaw removed

1. _____   7. _____

2. _____   8. _____

3. _____   9. _____

4. _____   10. _____

5. _____   11. _____

6. _____   12. _____

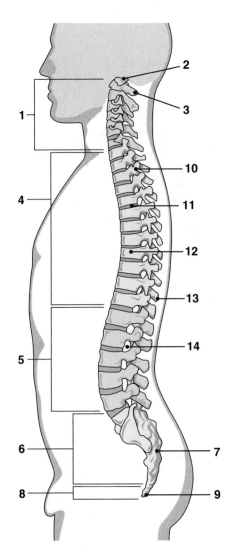

Vertebral column from the side

1. _____

2. _____

3. _____

4. _____

5. _____

6. _____

7. _____

8. _____

9. _____

10. _____

11. _____

12. _____

13. _____

14. _____

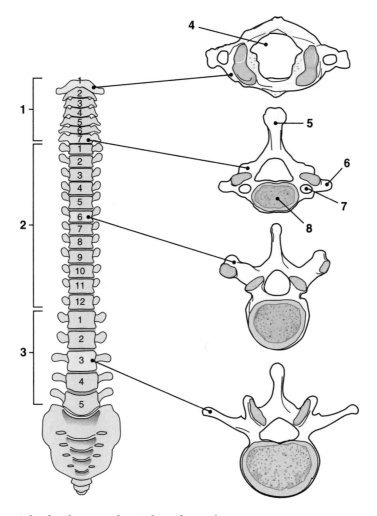

Front view of vertebral column and vertebrae from above

1. _____
2. _____
3. _____
4. _____

5. _____
6. _____
7. _____
8. _____

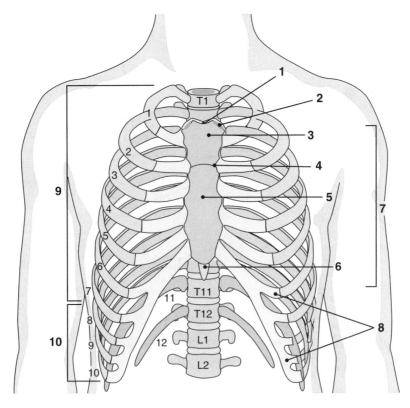

Bones of the thorax

1. _____

2. _____

3. _____

4. _____

5. _____

6. _____

7. _____

8. _____

9. _____

10. _____

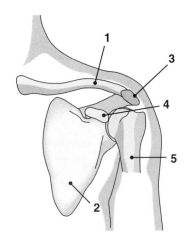

Bones of the shoulder girdle

1. _____

2. _____

3. _____

4. _____

5. _____

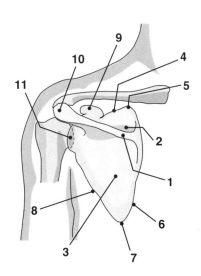

Left scapula (posterior view)

1. _____

2. _____

3. _____

4. _____

5. _____

6. _____

7. _____

8. _____

9. _____

10. _____

11. _____

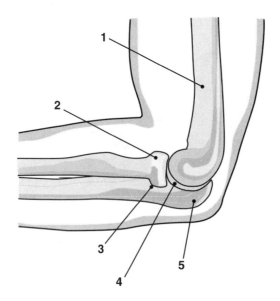

Lateral view of the right elbow

1. _____   4. _____

2. _____   5. _____

3. _____

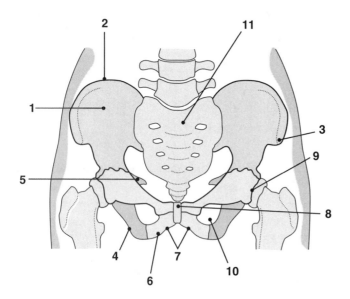

Pelvic bones, anterior view

1. _____

2. _____

3. _____

4. _____

5. _____

6. _____

7. _____

8. _____

9. _____

10. _____

11. _____

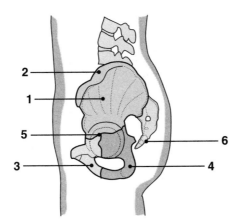

Pelvic bones, lateral view

1. _____   4. _____

2. _____   5. _____

3. _____   6. _____

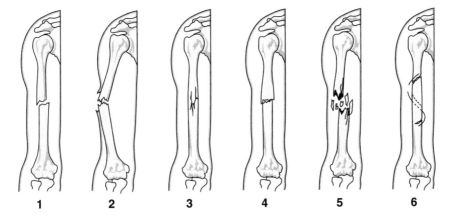

1	2	3	4	5	6

Types of fractures

1. _____   4. _____

2. _____   5. _____

3. _____   6. _____

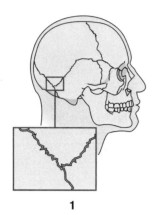

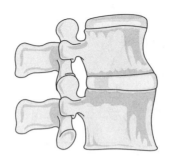

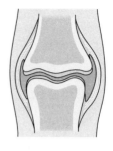

1	2	3

Types of joints

1. _____

2. _____

3. _____

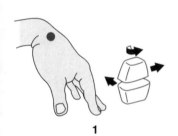

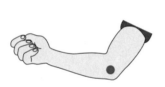

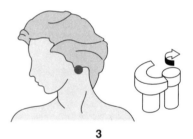

1	2	3

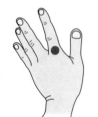

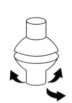

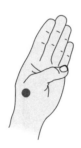

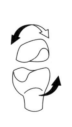

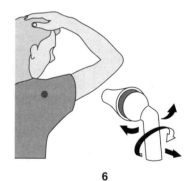

4	5	6

Types of synovial joints

1. _____   4. _____

2. _____   5. _____

3. _____   6. _____

VI. True–False

For each question, write T for true or F for false in the blank to the left of each number. If a statement is false, correct it by replacing the underlined term and write the correct statement in the blanks below the question.

_____ 1. The zygomatic bone is part of the <u>axial</u> skeleton.

_____

_____

_____ 2. The patella is part of the <u>axial</u> skeleton.

_____

_____

_____ 3. The mastoid process is part of the <u>frontal bone</u>.

_____

_____

_____ 4. There are <u>seven</u> pairs of true ribs.

_____

_____

_____ 5. In the anatomic position, the radius is <u>medial</u> to the ulna.

_____

_____

_____ 6. The shaft of a long bone is the <u>epiphysis</u>.

_____

_____

_____ 7. In a newborn infant, the entire vertebral column is <u>concave</u>.

_____

_____

_____ 8. The cervical curve is a <u>secondary</u> curve of the spine.

_____

_____

_____ 9. The palm is turned up or forward in <u>pronation</u>.

_____

_____

_____ 10. During development, transformation of cartilage into bone begins at the center of the <u>diaphysis</u>.

_____

_____

_____ 11. Movement of a part away from the midline of the body is termed <u>abduction</u>.

_____

_____

VII. Completion Exercise

Write the word or phrase that correctly completes each sentence.

1. When bone-forming cells mature and become enclosed in hardened bone material, they are referred to as _____

2. In the embryonic stage of bone development, most of the developing bones are made of _____

3. When bone is resorbed, cells that break down bone become active; these cells are called _____

4. The type of bone tissue that makes up the shaft of a long bone is called _____

5. The skull, vertebrae, ribs, and sternum make up the division of the skeleton called the _____

6. The os coxae is a fused bone consisting of the ilium, ischium, and _____

7. A suture is an example of an immovable joint also called a(n) _____

8. Pivot, hinge, and gliding joints are examples of freely movable joints also called _____

9. Swimming the overhead crawl requires a broad circular movement at the shoulder that is a combination of simpler movements. This combined motion is called

_____

10. When a toe dancer points her toes downward and flexes the arch of her foot, the motion is technically called

_____

VIII. Practical Applications

Study each discussion. Then write the appropriate word or phrase in the space provided.

Group A

A group of high school seniors was involved in a serious traffic accident on the way home from the prom.

1. There was a pronounced swelling of the upper right side of Michelle's head. X-ray films showed a fracture of the bone that forms the top and side of the cranium. This bone is the

_____

2. Michelle also suffered an injury to one of the two large bones of the pelvic girdle. This bone articulates with the sacrum and is named the

_____

3. Jason suffered multiple injuries to his left lower extremity. Protruding through the skin was a splintered portion of the longest bone in the body, the

_____

4. Susan thought her injuries were the least serious, so she walked several blocks to find help. Then she noticed that her right knee was not functioning normally. Examination revealed a fractured kneecap. The scientific name for the kneecap is

_____

5. Glen, the driver of the car, was forcibly thrown against the wheel. He suffered fractures of the sixth and seventh ribs, which are the last ribs in the group called the

_____

Group B

On his morning office schedule, Dr. J, an orthopedist (specialist in musculoskeletal disorders), was scheduled to see the following patients:

1. Mr. C, 48 years of age, who complained of severe pain of the great toe, as well as pain, swelling, redness, and inflammation of several joints of the foot and ankle. The primary care physician had noted on the referral that the patient had an elevated blood uric acid level. Dr. J performed an arthrocentesis (aspiration of joint fluid) of the metatarsophalangeal joint which showed uric acid crystals. This confirmed the diagnosis of

_____

2. Mrs. A, age 63, was evaluated for replacement of her right knee, which was almost immobile due to damage by osteoarthritis. Dr. J reviewed the radiographs, which showed a small joint space, abnormal bone deposits, and spurs preventing movement at the joint. The knee is an example of a freely movable joint, also called a(n) _____

3. Ashley, age 11, was seen by referral from the school nurse. The x-ray report stated an abnormality of 60-degree lateral curve of the thoracic spine. The physician diagnosed the abnormal lateral curvature of the spine as _____

Group C

Mrs. C, age 36, visited her physician's office because of swelling and pain in the joints of her hands and fingers. Examination revealed the following:

1. Evidence of inflammation and overgrowth of the membrane lining the joint cavities, a membrane that is called the _____

2. Difficulty in moving the joints of the fingers due to damage to the normally smooth tissue on the joint surface. This layer is called the _____

3. That Mrs. C was probably suffering from the common disorder called _____

IX. Short Essays

1. Explain why bone is described as living tissue.

_____

_____

_____

2. Describe the four curves of the adult spine and explain the purpose of these curves.

_____

_____

_____

3. Describe the structures that strengthen and stabilize a freely movable joint.

_____

_____

_____

Chapter

8

The Muscular System

I. Overview

There are three basic types of muscle tissue: *skeletal*, *smooth*, and *cardiac*. The focus of this chapter is skeletal muscle, which is attached to bones. Skeletal muscle is also called voluntary muscle, because normally it is under conscious control. The muscular system is composed of more than 650 individual muscles.

Skeletal muscles are activated by electrical impulses from the nervous system. A nerve fiber makes contact with a muscle cell at the *neuromuscular junction.* From this point, the impulse spreads along the muscle cell membrane, producing an electrical change called the *action potential.* As a result of this electrical change in the cells, the muscle can contract (shorten) to produce movement.

Muscle contraction occurs by the sliding together of filaments within the cell made of proteins called *actin* and *myosin.* These filaments make contact only in the presence of calcium, which is released from the endoplasmic reticulum of the muscle cell when the action potential spreads along the cell membrane. *ATP* is the direct source of energy for the contraction. To manufacture ATP, the cell must have adequate supplies of glucose and oxygen delivered by the blood. A reserve supply of glucose is stored in muscle cells in the form of a compound called *glycogen.* Additional oxygen is stored by a pigment in the cells called *myoglobin.*

When muscles do not receive enough oxygen, as during strenuous activity, they can produce a small amount of ATP and continue to function for a short period. As a result, however, the cells produce lactic acid, which eventually causes muscle fatigue. A person must then rest and continue to breathe in oxygen, which is used to convert the lactic acid into other substances. The amount of oxygen needed for this purpose is referred to as the *oxygen debt.*

Muscles usually work in groups to execute a body movement. The muscle that produces a given movement is called the *prime mover;* the muscle that produces the opposite action is the *antagonist.*

Muscles act with the bones of the skeleton as *lever systems,* in which the joint is the pivot point or *fulcrum.* Exercise and proper body mechanics help in maintaining muscle health and effectiveness. Continued activity delays the undesirable effects of aging.

II. Topics for Review

A. General characteristics of muscles
B. The mechanism of skeletal muscle contraction
    1. The energy for muscle contraction
    2. Effects of exercise
C. Muscle movement
    1. Muscle attachments
    2. Body mechanics
D. The muscular system
    1. Muscles of the head and the neck
    2. Muscles of the upper extremities
    3. Muscles of the trunk
    4. Muscles of the lower extremities
E. Disorders of muscles

III. Matching Exercises

Matching only within each group, write the answers in the spaces provided.

Group A

isotonic	contractility	excitability
neuromuscular junction	action potential	tonus
isometric		

1. The capacity of a muscle fiber to transmit electrical current _____

2. The point where a motor nerve fiber contacts a muscle cell _____

3. The electrical charge transmitted along the muscle cell membrane after stimulation _____

4. Term for muscle contractions in which the tone remains constant while the muscle shortens _____

5. The capacity of a muscle fiber to undergo shortening _____

6. The normal partially contracted state of muscles _____

7. Term for muscle contractions in which there is a great increase in muscle tension without change in muscle length _____

Group B

myoglobin	ATP	calcium
lactic acid	glycogen	actin

1. The compound that stores oxygen in muscle cells _____

2. The ion that must be released into the muscle cell before contraction _____

3. A protein filament needed for contraction in muscle cells _____

4. The substance that accumulates in muscles working without enough oxygen _____

5. The immediate source of energy for muscle contraction _____

6. The compound that stores glucose in muscle cells _____

Group C

origin	myosin	prime mover
vasodilation	antagonist	insertion

1. Name for the muscle that must relax during a given movement _____

2. The muscle attachment joined to a moving part of the body _____

3. Widening of a blood vessel _____

4. The muscle attachment joined to a more fixed part of the body _____

5. A protein needed for contraction in muscle cells _____

6. The muscle that produces a given movement _____

Group D

triceps brachii   pectoralis major   deltoid
latissimus dorsi   trapezius   biceps brachii
sternocleidomastoid

1. A triangular muscle over the back and neck that moves the shoulder _____

2. A muscle on the side of the neck that flexes the head on the chest _____

3. The muscle of the middle and lower back that is a powerful extensor of the arm (at the shoulder) _____

4. The muscle capping the shoulder and upper arm _____

5. A muscle on the front of the arm that acts as a flexor of the elbow and a supinator of the hand _____

6. The large muscle of the upper chest that flexes the arm across the body _____

7. The large muscle on the back of the arm that extends the elbow, as when delivering a blow _____

Group E

rotator cuff   levator ani   deep fascia
aponeurosis   tendon   diaphragm
torticollis   gastrocnemius

1. A cordlike structure that attaches a muscle to bone _____

2. A connective tissue sheath enclosing an entire muscle _____

3. The chief muscle of the calf of the leg _____

4. The muscle of the pelvic floor that aids in defecation _____

5. The chief muscle of respiration _____

6. A sheet of connective tissue that attaches certain muscles to bone or other muscles _____

7. A condition that may be caused by injury or spasm of a sternomastoid muscle

_____

8. A muscle group that supports the shoulder joint

_____

Group F

intercostal   sacrospinalis   gluteus maximus
buccinator   sartorius   iliopsoas
quadriceps femoris

1. The muscle that extends the leg at the knee, as in kicking a ball

_____

2. The longest muscle of the spine

_____

3. The muscle that forms much of the fleshy part of the buttock

_____

4. Muscles located between the ribs that aid in respiration

_____

5. The powerful flexor of the thigh

_____

6. The muscle that forms the fleshy part of the cheek

_____

7. The thin muscle that travels down and across the medial surface of the thigh

_____

Group G

bursitis   myositis   atrophy
ptosis   muscular dystrophy   myalgia

1. A group of disorders, seen more frequently in male children, that causes progressive weakness and paralysis

_____

2. A drooping of the eyelids, a common early symptom of myasthenia

_____

3. A term that means muscular pain

_____

4. Inflammation of a fluid-filled sac near a bone

_____

5. A wasting or decrease in the size of a muscle, usually from lack of activity

_____

6. Acute inflammation of muscle tissue

_____

IV. Multiple Choice

Select the best answer and write the letter of your choice in the blank.

1. A sudden and painful involuntary contraction of a muscle is called a

    a. strain
    b. sprain
    c. spasm
    d. fibrositis
    e. carpal tunnel syndrome

    1. _____

2. The lateral muscle of the leg that turns the sole of the foot outward (eversion) is the

    a. peroneus longus
    b. internal oblique
    c. extensor carpi
    d. teres minor
    e. adductor longus

    2. _____

3. Which of the following statements is *not* true of skeletal muscle?

    a. The cells are long and threadlike.
    b. It is normally under conscious control.
    c. It is described as striated.
    d. The cells are multinucleated.
    e. It is involuntary.

    3. _____

4. When muscles and bones act together in the body as a lever system, the pivot point or fulcrum of the system is the

    a. joint
    b. tendon
    c. extensor
    d. myoglobin
    e. levator

    4. _____

5. The hamstring muscles act to

    a. extend the leg
    b. flex the leg
    c. abduct the thigh
    d. adduct the arm
    e. move the hand

    5. _____

6. Student's elbow and housemaid's knee are examples of

    a. cramps
    b. seizures
    c. bunions
    d. bursitis
    e. tendinitis

    6. _____

V. Labeling

For each of the following illustrations, write the name or names of each labeled part on the numbered lines.

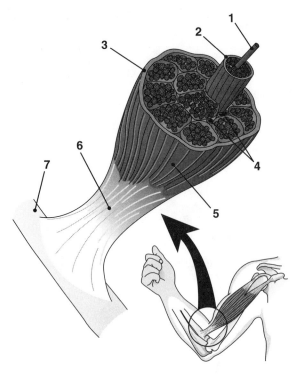

Structure of a skeletal muscle

1. _____   5. _____

2. _____   6. _____

3. _____   7. _____

4. _____

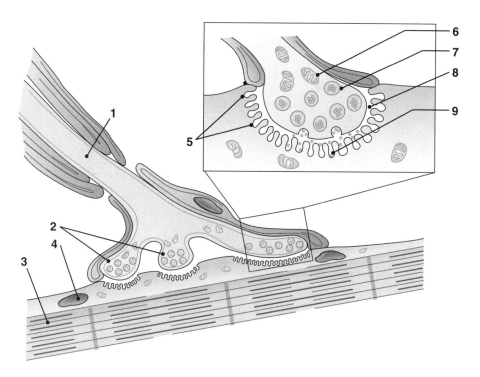

Neuromuscular junction

1. _____

2. _____

3. _____

4. _____

5. _____

6. _____

7. _____

8. _____

9. _____

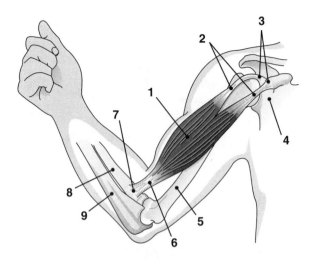

Diagram of a muscle showing three attachments to bones

1. _____

2. _____

3. _____

4. _____

5. _____

6. _____

7. _____

8. _____

9. _____

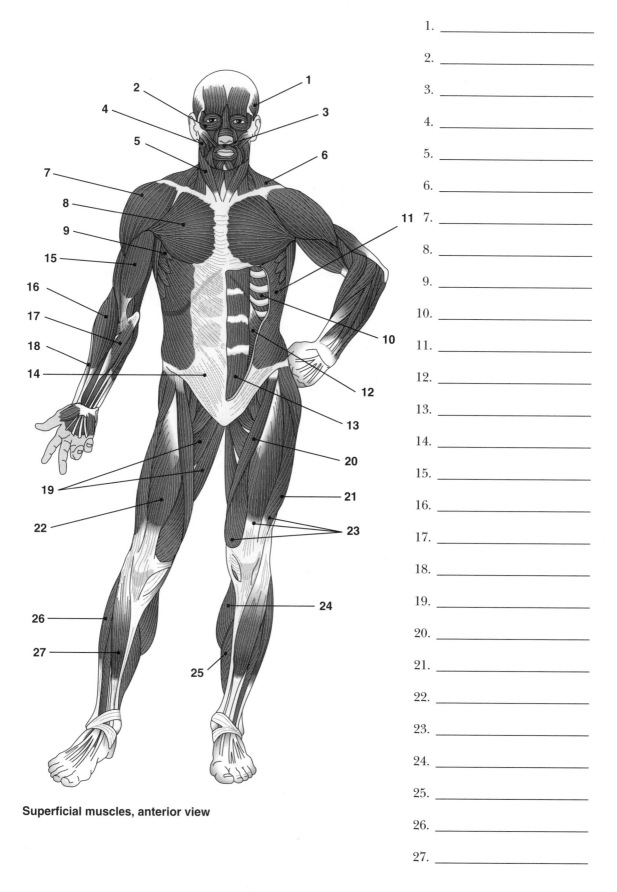

Superficial muscles, anterior view

1. _____

2. _____

3. _____

4. _____

5. _____

6. _____

7. _____

8. _____

9. _____

10. _____

11. _____

12. _____

13. _____

14. _____

15. _____

16. _____

17. _____

18. _____

19. _____

20. _____

21. _____

22. _____

23. _____

24. _____

25. _____

26. _____

27. _____

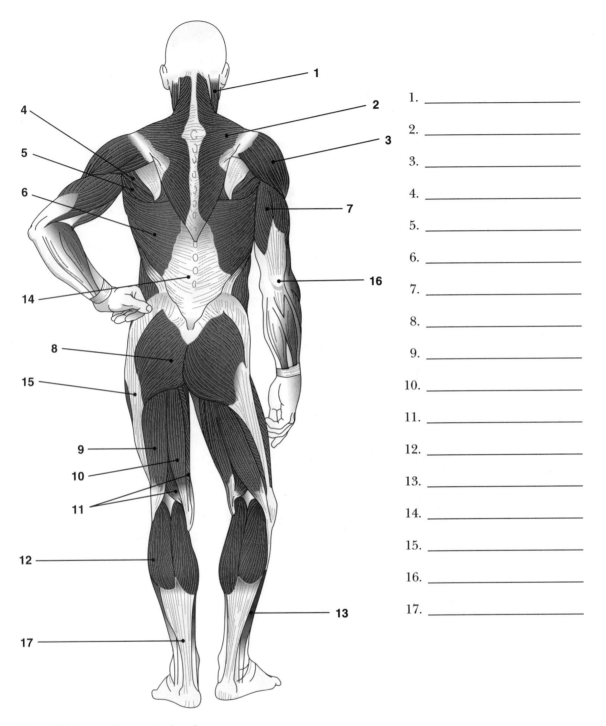

Superficial muscles, posterior view

1. _____
2. _____
3. _____
4. _____
5. _____
6. _____
7. _____
8. _____
9. _____
10. _____
11. _____
12. _____
13. _____
14. _____
15. _____
16. _____
17. _____

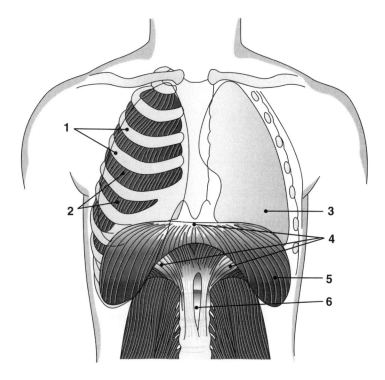

The diaphragm

1. _____   4. _____

2. _____   5. _____

3. _____   6. _____

VI. True–False

For each question, write T for true or F for false in the blank to the left of each number. If a statement is false, correct it by replacing the underlined term and write the correct statement in the blanks below the question.

_____ 1. Muscles enter into oxygen debt when they are functioning anaerobically.

_____

_____

_____ 2. Actin is the light filament in skeletal muscle cells.

_____

_____

_____ 3. In an isotonic contraction, muscle tension increases but the muscle does not shorten.

_____

_____

_____ 4. The internal abdominal oblique forms the middle layer of the abdominal wall.

_____

_____

_____ 5. The origin of a muscle is attached to a part of the body that the muscle puts into action.

_____

_____

_____ 6. The triceps brachii flexes the arm at the elbow.

_____

_____

_____ 7. The intercostal muscles are between the ribs.

_____

_____

_____ 8. The flexor carpi and extensor carpi muscles move the <u>foot.</u>

_____

_____

VII. Completion Exercise

Write the word or phrase that correctly completes each sentence.

1. Normally, muscles are in a partially contracted state, even though they are not in use at the time. This state of mild constant tension is called

    _____

2. A movement is initiated by a muscle or set of muscles called the

    _____

3. The less movable (more fixed) attachment of a muscle is the

    _____

4. The muscle of the lips is the

    _____

5. Muscles functioning without enough oxygen will fatigue as a result of the accumulation of

    _____

6. The muscle attachment that is usually relatively fixed is called its

    _____

7. The movement of a prime mover is opposed by a muscle or set of muscles called the

    _____

8. A group of muscles that covers the front and sides of the femur and extends the leg is the

    _____

9. There are four pairs of muscles for chewing. The muscle located at the angle of the jaw is called the

    _____

10. The muscles of the pelvic floor together form the

    _____

11. A superficial muscle of the neck and upper back acts at the shoulder. This muscle is the

    _____

12. The muscle on the front of the leg that raises the sole of the foot (dorsiflexion) is the

    _____

13. The muscular partition between the thoracic and abdominal cavities is the

    _____

14. The band of connective tissue that attaches the gastrocnemius muscle to the heel is the

    _____

VIII. Practical Applications

Study each discussion. Then write the appropriate word or phrase in the space provided.

Group A

Driver J and his three companions tried to race an oncoming train to an intersection. J misjudged the speed of the train, and the train crashed into the car. All four occupants of the car received multiple injuries.

1. Driver J was thrown against the steering wheel, which punctured his chest. This puncture involved the muscles between the ribs, called the _____

2. Mr. K, the occupant sitting next to the driver, suffered facial injuries in which the muscle that encircles the eye was cut. This muscle is called the _____

3. Ms. L was thrown out of the car and received lacerations and fractures of the lower extremities, including the calf of the leg. The largest muscle of the leg is the _____

4. Mr. M received shoulder and upper back lacerations. They involved the muscle that covers the shoulder and abducts the arm, the _____

Group B

In the outpatient physical therapy department, the following patients were seen for their exercise programs.

1. Mrs. K had suffered a stroke that produced weakness of the left lower extremity. Today, she was learning exercises to strengthen the large muscle used in standing that forms most of the buttock. This muscle is the _____

2. Mr. P was recovering from an injury to the upper arm that required surgery to repair damaged muscle and a long period of immobility. Now, he was receiving exercise to strengthen the large extensor muscle of the elbow located in the dorsal part of the arm. This muscle is the _____

3. Ms. R, age 68, was seen for exercises to increase the strength of the long extensor muscle of the back. Her history included a healed compression fracture of the lumbar vertebrae that resulted from a fall. The muscle that holds the spine erect is the _____

4. Sara was recuperating from a knee injury sustained while snow skiing. She was receiving ultrasound treatments to reduce pain in the joint and exercises to strengthen muscles across the knee. The muscle in the anterior thigh that extends the leg is the _____

5. Sara was also given exercises to strengthen the group of muscles in the posterior thigh that flex the leg. This group of muscles in known as the _____

IX. Short Essays

1. Compare the location and function of the three types of muscle tissue.

   _____

   _____

   _____

2. List the requirements for skeletal muscle contraction and explain the role of each.

   _____

   _____

   _____

3. Briefly describe what happens in muscle cells functioning anaerobically.

   _____

   _____

   _____

Unit IV

COORDINATION AND CONTROL

9

The Nervous System: The Spinal Cord and Spinal Nerves

I. Overview

The nervous system is the body's coordinating system, receiving, sorting, and controlling responses to both internal and external changes (stimuli). The nervous system as a whole is divided structurally into the *central nervous system* (*CNS*), made up of the brain and the spinal cord, and the *peripheral nervous system* (*PNS*), made up of the cranial and spinal nerves, which connects all parts of the body with the central nervous system. The brain and cranial nerves are the subject of Chapter 10. Functionally, the nervous system is divided into the somatic (voluntary) system and autonomic (involuntary) system, which is also known as the visceral nervous system.

The nervous system functions by means of the *nerve impulse,* an electrical current or *action potential* that spreads along the membrane of the *neuron* (nerve cell). Each neuron is composed of a cell body and nerve fibers, which are thread-like extensions from the cell body. A *dendrite* is a fiber that carries impulses toward the cell body, and an *axon* is a fiber that carries impulses away from the cell body. Some axons are covered with a sheath of fatty material called *myelin,* which insulates the fiber and speeds conduction along the fiber. In the PNS, nerve cell fibers are collected in bundles to form *nerves.* Bundles of fibers in the CNS are called *tracts.*

Nerve cells make contact at a junction called a *synapse.* Here, a nerve impulse travels across a very narrow cleft between the cells by means of a chemical referred to as a *neurotransmitter.* Neurotransmitters are released from axons of presynaptic cells to be picked up by receptors in the membranes of responding cells, the postsynaptic cells.

A neuron may be classified as either a sensory (afferent) type, which carries impulses toward the central nervous system, or a motor (efferent) type, which carries impulses away from the central nervous system. *Interneurons* are connecting neurons within the central nervous system.

The basic functional pathway of the nervous system is a *reflex arc,* in which an impulse travels from a receptor, along a sensory neuron to a synapse or synapses in the central nervous system, and then along a motor neuron to an effector organ that carries out a response. The spinal cord carries impulses to and from the brain. It is also a center for simple reflex activities in which responses are coordinated within the cord.

The *autonomic nervous system* controls unconscious activities. This system regulates the actions of glands, smooth muscle, and the heart muscle. The autonomic nervous system has two divisions, the *sympathetic nervous system* and the *parasympathetic nervous system,* which generally have opposite effects on a given organ.

II. Topics for Review

A. Anatomic divisions of the nervous system
  1. Central nervous system
  2. Peripheral nervous system
B. Functional divisions of the nervous system
  1. Somatic (voluntary)
  2. Autonomic (involuntary)
C. Neuroglia
D. Neurons and their functions
  1. Fibers
  2. Myelin sheath
  3. Types of neurons

4. Types of nerves
5. The nerve impulse
6. The synapse
7. The reflex arc
E. Spinal cord
1. Location
2. Structure
3. Functions
4. Simple reflexes
5. Disorders involving the spinal cord
F. Spinal nerves
1. Location and structure
2. Branches
3. Disorders
G. Autonomic nervous system
1. Divisions
a. Sympathetic
b. Parasympathetic
2. Functions

III. Matching Exercises

Matching only within each group, write the answers in the spaces provided.

Group A

tract   neuron   nerve impulse
dendrite   root   plexus
synapse   axon

1. An electrical charge that spreads along the membrane of a
   nerve cell   _____

2. A nerve cell fiber that carries impulses away from the cell body   _____

3. The scientific name for a nerve cell   _____

4. A network formed by the larger anterior branches of a
   spinal nerve   _____

5. A branch of a spinal nerve that attaches to the spinal cord   _____

6. The point at which impulses are transmitted from one
   nerve cell to another   _____

7. The part of a neuron that receives a stimulus   _____

8. A bundle of neuron fibers within the CNS   _____

Group B

action potential   neurilemma   parasympathetic system
reflex arc   ganglion   sensory
sympathetic system

1. Another name for a nerve impulse _____

2. Term for neurons that carry impulses toward the CNS _____

3. A collection of neuron cell bodies located outside the CNS _____

4. The sheath around some neuron fibers that aids in regeneration _____

5. The system that promotes the fight-or-flight response _____

6. The system that stimulates the digestive and urinary tracts _____

7. A complete pathway through the nervous system from stimulus to response _____

Group C

craniosacral	reflex	neurotransmitter
thoracolumbar	neuroglia	efferent
nerve	mixed	

1. Term that describes the sympathetic portion of the autonomic nervous system, based on where it originates _____

2. Term that describes most nerves, notably the spinal nerves, because they contain both afferent and efferent fibers _____

3. A simple, automatic response that involves few neurons _____

4. A chemical that carries an impulse across a synapse _____

5. Term that describes the parasympathetic portion of the autonomic nervous system, based on where it originates _____

6. A term that means the same as *motor* _____

7. A bundle of nerve cell fibers located outside the central nervous system _____

8. Connective tissue cells of the nervous system _____

Group D

stretch reflex	brachial plexus	sciatic nerve
motor neurons	peripheral neuritis	cervical plexus
interneuron	sensory fibers	

1. The network of nerves that supplies the upper extremities _____

2. Degeneration of nerves supplying the extremities _____

3. A neuron that relays information within the CNS _____

4. The type of response exemplified by the knee jerk _____

5. The network of nerves that supplies the neck muscles _____

6. The type of cells in the ventral gray horn of the spinal cord _____

7. The largest branch of the lumbosacral plexus _____

8. The structures contained in the dorsal root of a spinal nerve _____

Group E

sympathetic chain   acetylcholine   shingles
adrenal   adrenergic   visceral
paraplegia

1. The gland that produces epinephrine _____

2. The common name for herpes zoster, a viral disease of nerves _____

3. The neurotransmitter released from neurons of the parasympathetic nervous system _____

4. A cordlike strand of ganglia that extends along the spinal column _____

5. Loss of sensation and motion in the lower part of the body _____

6. Another term for the autonomic nervous system _____

7. Adjective for a response activated by the neurotransmitter epinephrine _____

IV. Multiple Choice

Select the best answer and write the letter of your choice in the blank.

1. A sudden electrical change that spreads along a nerve cell membrane is called a(n)   1. _____

   a. dendrite
   b. neurilemma
   c. action potential
   d. receptor
   e. effector

2. Which of the following are effectors of the nervous system?   2. _____

   a. sensory neurons and ganglia
   b. receptors and neurotransmitters
   c. synapses and dendrites
   d. adipose tissue and tendons
   e. muscles and glands

3. Which of the following substances is a neurotransmitter? 3. _____

   a. melanin
   b. acetylcholine
   c. sebum
   d. myelin
   e. actin

4. Myelinated fibers are found in the 4. _____

   a. dorsal horn
   b. ventral horn
   c. central canal
   d. white matter
   e. gray matter

5. Cell bodies of sensory neurons are collected in ganglia located on each 5. _____

   a. dorsal root
   b. sympathetic chain
   c. ventral root
   d. effector organ
   e. plexus

6. Sensory nerves are also described as 6. _____

   a. afferent
   b. sensory
   c. tracts
   d. ascending
   e. efferent

7. The voluntary nervous system controls 7. _____

   a. smooth muscle
   b. skeletal muscle
   c. glands
   d. cardiac muscle
   e. visceral muscle

V. Labeling

For each of the following illustrations, write the name or names of each labeled part on the numbered lines.

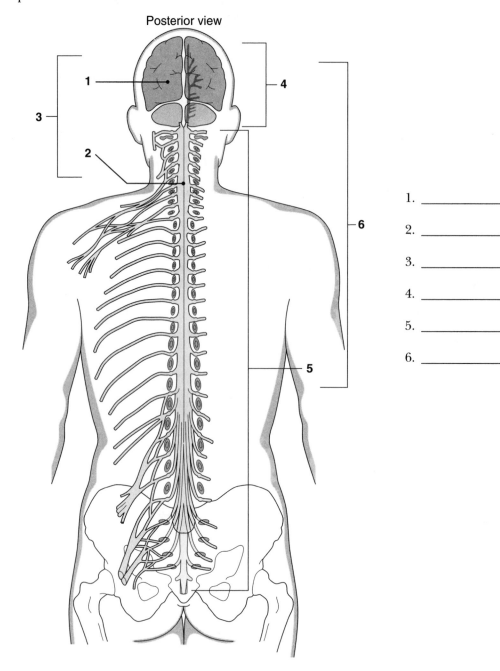

Posterior view

Anatomic divisions of the nervous system

1. _____

2. _____

3. _____

4. _____

5. _____

6. _____

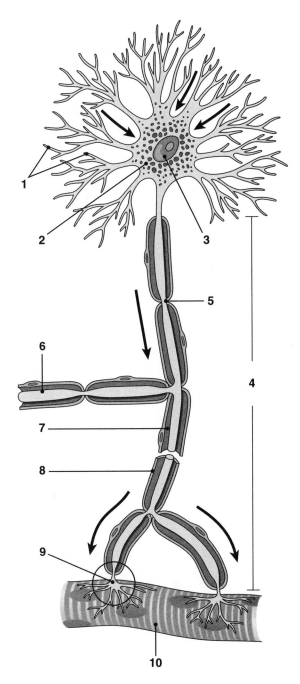

Diagram of a motor neuron

1. _____

2. _____

3. _____

4. _____

5. _____

6. _____

7. _____

8. _____

9. _____

10. _____

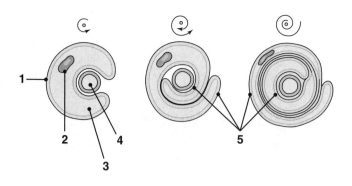

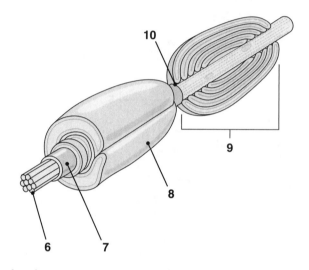

Formation of a myelin sheath

1. _____

2. _____

3. _____

4. _____

5. _____

6. _____

7. _____

8. _____

9. _____

10. _____

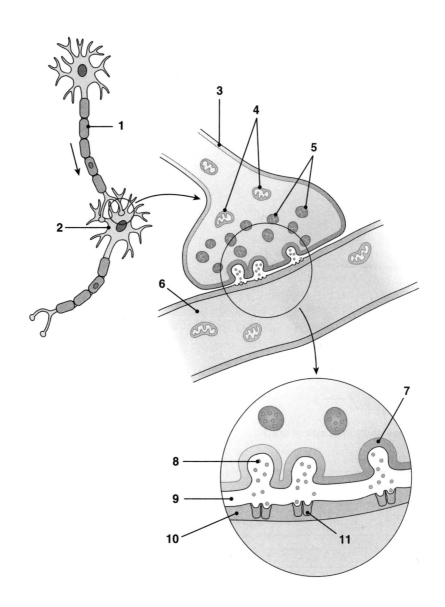

A synapse

1. _____

2. _____

3. _____

4. _____

5. _____

6. _____

7. _____

8. _____

9. _____

10. _____

11. _____

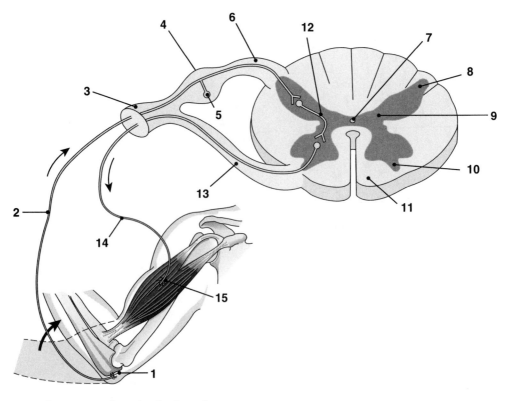

Reflex arc and cross section of spinal cord

1. _____
2. _____
3. _____
4. _____
5. _____
6. _____
7. _____
8. _____

9. _____
10. _____
11. _____
12. _____
13. _____
14. _____
15. _____

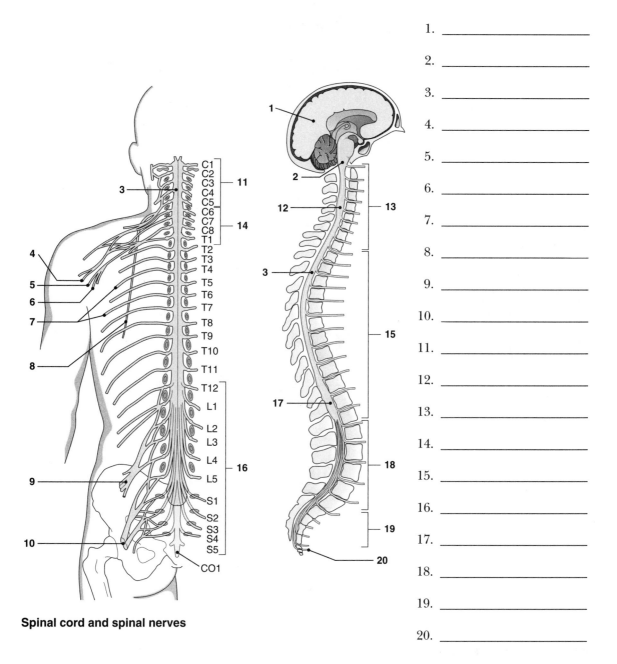

C1
C2
C3
C4
C5
C6
C7
C8
T1
T2
T3
T4
T5
T6
T7
T8
T9
T10
T11
T12
L1
L2
L3
L4
L5
S1
S2
S3
S4
S5
CO1

Spinal cord and spinal nerves

1. _____

2. _____

3. _____

4. _____

5. _____

6. _____

7. _____

8. _____

9. _____

10. _____

11. _____

12. _____

13. _____

14. _____

15. _____

16. _____

17. _____

18. _____

19. _____

20. _____

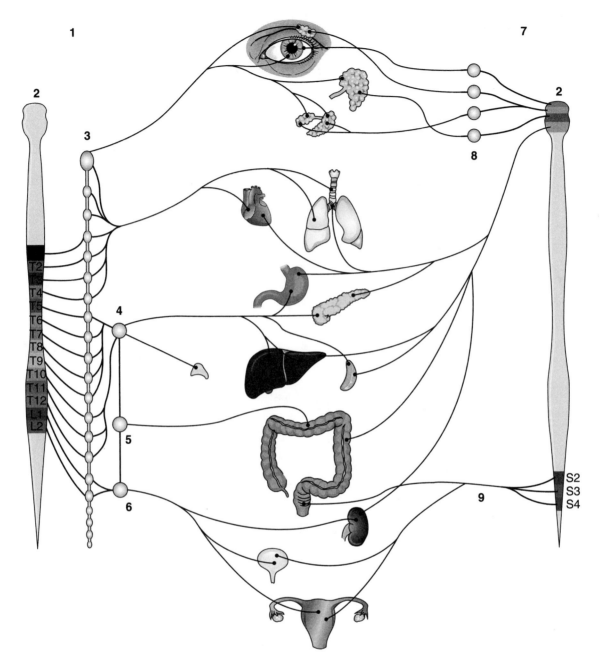

Autonomic nervous system

1. _____

2. _____

3. _____

4. _____

5. _____

6. _____

7. _____

8. _____

9. _____

VI. True–False

For each question, write T for true or F for false in the blank to the left of each number. If a statement is false, correct it by replacing the underlined term and write the correct statement in the blanks below the question.

_____ 1. Motor nerves are also described as <u>afferent.</u>

_____

_____

_____ 2. The cranial and spinal nerves make up the <u>peripheral</u> nervous system.

_____

_____

_____ 3. The <u>somatic</u> nervous system is the voluntary nervous system.

_____

_____

_____ 4. Unmyelinated fibers form the <u>gray</u> matter of the nervous system.

_____

_____

_____ 5. A <u>sensory</u> neuron carries impulses away from the central nervous system.

_____

_____

_____ 6. A <u>tract</u> is a bundle of neuron fibers within the central nervous system.

_____

_____

_____ 7. An <u>axon</u> carries nerve impulses toward the cell body.

_____

_____

_____ 8. Sensory impulses enter the <u>dorsal</u> horn of the spinal cord.

_____

_____

_____ 9. The <u>parasympathetic system</u> has terminal ganglia.

_____

_____

_____ 10. The parasympathetic system is <u>adrenergic.</u>

_____

_____

_____ 11. At a synapse, neurotransmitter is released from the <u>postsynaptic cell.</u>

_____

_____

VII. Completion Exercise

Write the word or phrase that correctly completes each sentence.

1. A nerve cell is also called a(n) _____

2. The brain and spinal cord together are referred to as the _____

3. The fatty material that covers some axons is called _____

4. The junction between two neurons is a(n) _____

5. The connective tissue cells of the nervous system are _____

6. A chemical released at a synapse is a(n) _____

7. Dilation of the bronchial tubes is increased by the part of the autonomic nervous system called the _____

8. The network of spinal nerves that supplies the pelvis and legs is the _____

9. A specialized nerve ending that can detect a stimulus is a(n) _____

10. The small channel in the center of the spinal cord that contains cerebrospinal fluid is the _____

11. A neuron fiber that conducts impulses away from the cell body is a(n) _____

VIII. Practical Applications

Study each discussion. Then write the appropriate word or phrase in the space provided.

1. Ms. B was being treated for lung cancer. Her symptoms included pain in the back and weakness of the right arm. X-ray studies showed a tumor encroaching on the space containing the spinal cord. This space is called the

   _____

2. Mr. C was involved in a serious automobile accident. A study of shoulder radiographs showed a fractured humerus that cut into the network of nerves that supplies the upper extremity. This mass of nerves is called the

   _____

3. Mr. W, a patient with diabetes mellitus for 10 years, complained of pain and numbness of his feet. In observing Mr. W walk, the physician noted there was weakness in the muscles responsible for dorsiflexion of the foot. These symptoms are caused by a degenerative disorder of nerves to the extremities known as

   _____

4. Ms. D fell down a staircase. A diagnostic study of her injuries included the removal of fluid from the space below the end of the spinal cord. Because of the location of the needle insertion, this is called a(n)

   _____

5. Debra had sustained some lacerations on her hands and face and was waiting to have them repaired. She was noted to have rapid heart rate, elevated blood pressure, excess sweating, and dilated pupils. These symptoms indicate overactivity of one of the divisions of the nervous system known as the

   _____

IX. Short Essays

1. Describe a synapse between two neurons.

   _____
   _____
   _____

2. What are neuroglia, and what are some functions of neuroglia?

   _____
   _____
   _____

3. List three ways that neurotransmitters are removed from a synaptic cleft and cite the significance of the different methods.

   _____
   _____
   _____

4. Define a *reflex arc,* and list the components of a reflex arc.

   _____
   _____
   _____

The Nervous System: The Brain and Cranial Nerves

I. Overview

The brain consists of the two cerebral hemispheres, the diencephalon, the brain stem, and the cerebellum, each with specific functions.

The brain and spinal cord are covered by three layers of fibrous membranes called the *meninges.* Aiding in the protection of the brain and cord is the *cerebrospinal fluid,* which is produced by the choroid plexuses (capillary networks) in four ventricles (spaces) within the brain.

Connected with the brain are 12 pairs of *cranial nerves,* most of which supply structures in the head. Most of these, like all the spinal nerves, are mixed nerves containing both sensory and motor fibers. A few of the cranial nerves contain only sensory fibers, whereas others are motor in function.

II. Topics for Review

A. Protective structures of the CNS
    1. The meninges
    2. Cerebrospinal fluid
B. Divisions of the brain
    1. Cerebral hemispheres
       a. Lobes
       b. Cortex
    2. Diencephalon
       a. Thalamus
       b. Hypothalamus

3. Brain stem
   a. Midbrain
   b. Pons
   c. Medulla oblongata
4. Cerebellum
C. Brain studies
D. Disorders of the brain
E. Cranial nerves
   1. Disorders of the cranial nerves

III. Matching Exercises

Matching only within each group, write the answers in the spaces provided.

Group A

sulci	meninges	hemisphere
lobes	brain stem	ventricles
thalamus	gyri	cortex

1. The collective name for the three brain coverings   _____

2. The shallow grooves in the cortex of the cerebrum   _____

3. Each half of the cerebrum   _____

4. The region of the diencephalon that acts as a relay center for sensory stimuli   _____

5. Individual subdivisions of the cerebrum that regulate specific functions   _____

6. The spaces within the brain where cerebrospinal fluid (CSF) is produced   _____

7. The part of the brain composed of the midbrain, pons, and medulla   _____

8. The elevated portions of the cerebral cortex   _____

9. The thin layer of gray matter on the surface of the cerebrum   _____

Group B

dura mater   arachnoid   pia mater
meningitis   choroid plexus   subarachnoid space
arachnoid villi   hydrocephalus   glioma

1. The weblike middle meningeal layer   _____

2. A brain tumor derived from neuroglia   _____

3. A condition that may result from obstruction of the normal flow of CSF   _____

4. The innermost layer of the meninges, the delicate membrane in which there are many blood vessels   _____

5. The area in which cerebrospinal fluid collects before its return to the blood   _____

6. The vascular network in a ventricle that forms cerebrospinal fluid   _____

7. Inflammation of the coverings of the brain due to viruses or bacteria   _____

8. The projections in the dural sinuses through which CSF is returned to the blood   _____

9. The outermost layer of the meninges, which is the thickest and toughest   _____

Group C

medulla oblongata   occipital lobe   motor cortex
corpus callosum   cerebellum   temporal lobe
parietal lobe

1. The portion of the cerebral cortex where visual impulses from the retina are interpreted

_____

2. The division of the brain that coordinates voluntary muscles and helps to maintain balance

_____

3. A band of white matter that acts as a bridge between the cerebral hemispheres

_____

4. The part of the brain between the pons and the spinal cord

_____

5. The portion of the cerebral cortex where auditory impulses are interpreted

_____

6. The area in each frontal lobe, near the central sulcus, that controls the voluntary muscles

_____

7. Location of a sensory area for interpretation of pain, touch, and temperature

_____

Group D

diencephalon   central sulcus   lateral sulcus
internal capsule   limbic system   medulla oblongata

1. The groove that runs at right angles to the longitudinal fissure between the frontal and parietal lobes

_____

2. The portion of the brain that contains the thalamus and hypothalamus

_____

3. The location of the vasomotor center, which regulates smooth muscle contraction in blood vessels

_____

4. The groove that curves along the side of each hemisphere and separates the temporal lobe from the frontal and parietal lobes

_____

5. A crowded strip of nerve fibers that carries messages to and from the brain cortex

_____

6. The region consisting of portions of the cerebrum and diencephalon that is involved in emotional states and behavior

_____

Group E

encephalitis   epilepsy   neuralgia
aphasia   cerebrovascular accident   Parkinson's disease
cerebral palsy

1. A general term meaning nerve pain

_____

2. A chronic brain disorder that usually can be diagnosed by electroencephalography

_____

3. Damage to brain tissue caused by a blood clot, ruptured vessel, or embolism; a stroke

_____

4. Loss of the power of expression by speech or writing

_____

5. A congenital disorder characterized by muscle involvement ranging from weakness to paralysis

_____

6. A brain disorder that has been treated with the drug L-dopa

_____

7. The general term for inflammation of the brain

_____

Group F

trigeminal nerve   accessory nerve   vestibulocochlear nerve
optic nerve   hypoglossal nerve   oculomotor nerve
vagus nerve   olfactory nerve   facial nerve

1. The nerve that carries motor impulses to two neck muscles

_____

2. The sensory nerve that carries visual impulses

_____

3. The nerve that carries impulses for the sense of smell

_____

4. The nerve that supplies most of the organs in the thoracic and abdominal cavities

_____

5. The nerve that controls tongue muscles

_____

6. The nerve that supplies the muscles of facial expression

_____

7. The nerve with three branches that carries general sensory impulses from the face and head

_____

8. The nerve that contains sensory fibers for hearing

_____

9. The nerve that controls contraction of most eye muscles

_____

IV. Multiple Choice

Select the best answer and write the letter of your choice in the blank.

1. The pia mater is

    a. the innermost layer of the meninges
    b. the middle layer of the meninges
    c. the network of vessels that produces cerebrospinal fluid
    d. a raised area on the surface of the cerebrum
    e. the part of the brain that connects with the spinal cord

1. _____

2. Which of the following is *not* a lobe of the cerebrum?　　　　2. _____

   a. parietal
   b. frontal
   c. ventricular
   d. occipital
   e. temporal

3. The reticular formation is　　　　3. _____

   a. a venous channel in the brain
   b. a region of the limbic system that controls wakefulness and sleep
   c. a deep groove that divides the cerebral hemispheres
   d. the part of the temporal lobe concerned with the sense of smell
   e. the fifth lobe of the cerebrum

4. The part of the brain stem that contains relay centers for eye and　　　　4. _____
   ear reflexes is the

   a. cortex
   b. thalamus
   c. cerebellum
   d. midbrain
   e. cerebrum

5. Impulses for the sense of smell travel to the　　　　5. _____

   a. arachnoid
   b. cerebral aqueduct
   c. choroid plexus
   d. hippocampus
   e. olfactory bulbs

6. The glossopharyngeal nerve supplies the　　　　6. _____

   a. face and eye
   b. ear and pharynx
   c. ear and nose
   d. tongue and pharynx
   e. lower jaw and thoracic organs

7. Multi-infarct dementia is the result of　　　　7. _____

   a. accumulation of an abnormal protein
   b. ischemia (lack of blood supply)
   c. obstruction of the flow of CSF
   d. infection of the brain coverings
   e. lack of neurotransmitters

V. Labeling

For each of the following illustrations, write the name or names of each labeled part on the numbered lines.

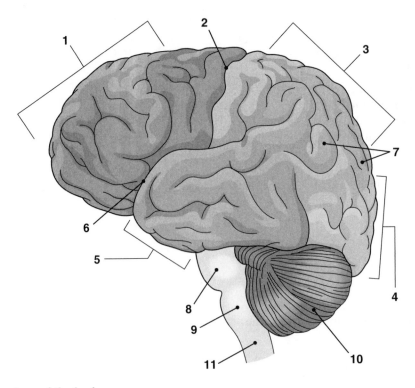

External surface of the brain

1. _____

2. _____

3. _____

4. _____

5. _____

6. _____

7. _____

8. _____

9. _____

10. _____

11. _____

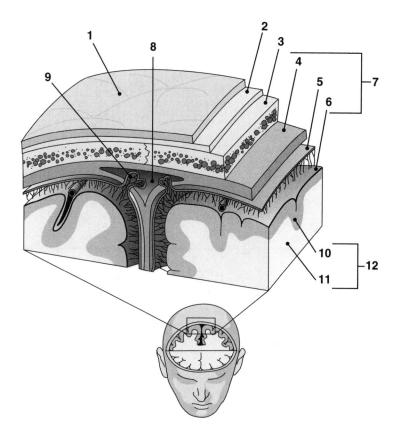

Frontal section of the top of the head

1. _____

2. _____

3. _____

4. _____

5. _____

6. _____

7. _____

8. _____

9. _____

10. _____

11. _____

12. _____

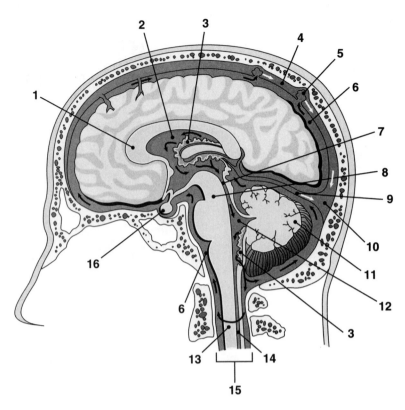

Flow of cerebrospinal fluid

1. _____

2. _____

3. _____

4. _____

5. _____

6. _____

7. _____

8. _____

9. _____

10. _____

11. _____

12. _____

13. _____

14. _____

15. _____

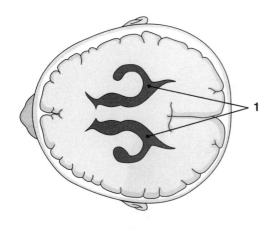

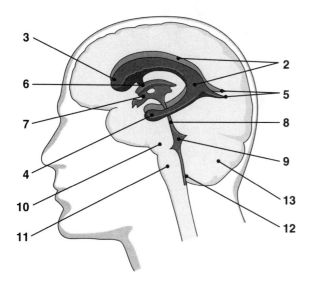

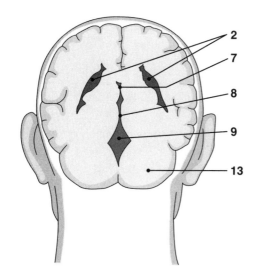

Ventricles of the brain

1. _____
2. _____
3. _____
4. _____
5. _____
6. _____
7. _____
8. _____
9. _____
10. _____
11. _____
12. _____
13. _____

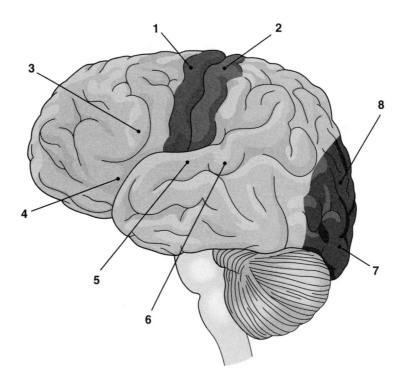

Functional areas of the cerebral cortex

1. _____

2. _____

3. _____

4. _____

5. _____

6. _____

7. _____

8. _____

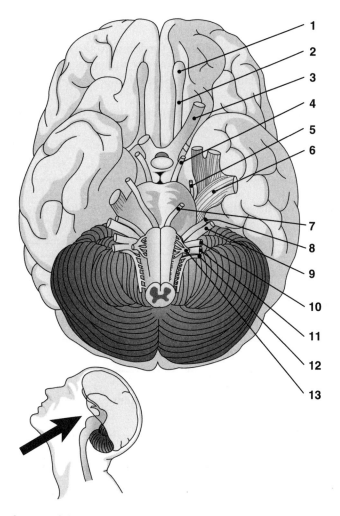

Base of the brain showing cranial nerves

1. _____

2. _____

3. _____

4. _____

5. _____

6. _____

7. _____

8. _____

9. _____

10. _____

11. _____

12. _____

13. _____

VI. True–False

For each question, write T for true or F for false in the blank to the left of each number. If a statement is false, correct it by replacing the underlined term and write the correct statement in the blanks below the question.

_____ 1. Most of the cranial nerves supply structures in the <u>head</u>.

_____

_____

_____ 2. The raised areas on the surface of the cerebrum are called <u>sulci</u>.

_____

_____

_____ 3. The <u>pia mater</u> is the outermost layer of the meninges.

_____

_____

_____ 4. The <u>pons</u> is the middle portion of the brain stem.

_____

_____

_____ 5. The visual area of the cerebral cortex is in the <u>occipital</u> lobe.

_____

_____

_____ 6. The area outside the dura mater is described as <u>subdural</u>.

_____

_____

_____ 7. The vestibulocochlear nerve (VIII) is a <u>sensory</u> nerve.

_____

_____

_____ 8. The trigeminal nerve is the <u>fifth</u> cranial nerve.

_____

_____

VII.   Completion Exercise

Write the word or phrase that correctly completes each sentence.

1. The largest part of the brain is the
    _____

2. The three layers of membranes that surround the brain and spinal cord are called the
    _____

3. The delicate innermost membrane surrounding the brain is the
    _____

4. The clear liquid that helps to support and protect the brain and spinal cord is
    _____

5. The number of pairs of cranial nerves is
    _____

6. A degenerative disorder of the cerebral cortex and hippocampus characterized by accumulation of amyloid (an abnormal protein) and tangling of neuron fibers is
    _____

7. The spinal cord connects with the part of the brain called the
    _____

8. The thin layer of gray matter that forms the surface of each cerebral hemisphere is the
    _____

9. Most brain tumors are derived from neuroglia and are called
    _____

10. The four chambers within the brain where cerebrospinal fluid is produced are the
    _____

11. The region of the diencephalon that helps maintain homeostasis (*eg,* water balance, appetite, and body temperature) and controls the autonomic nervous system is the
    _____

12. Any obstruction to the normal flow of CSF may give rise to increased fluid pressure and brain damage. This condition is called
    _____

13. Records of the electrical activity of the brain can be made with an instrument called a(n)
    _____

14. Except for the first two pairs, all the cranial nerves arise from the
    _____

VIII.   Practical Applications

Study each discussion. Then write the appropriate word or phrase in the space provided.

1. Mrs. N, age 67, had been found lying on the floor, unconscious. She had a history of hypertension and was diagnosed as having had a stroke. Now, she is unable to speak or write. This loss of ability to communicate through language is called _____

2. Mr. H, age 42, had been suffering from severe headaches for 8 weeks. A brain study involving three-dimensional x-ray images was ordered. Such a study is called a(n) _____

3. Young A, age 10, was brought to the emergency room after he had fallen from his bicycle and hit his head, resulting in external bleeding. Studies were done to determine the possibility of internal damage due to a tear in the wall of a dural sinus. Such a tear causes a lesion filled with blood, known as a(n) _____

4. Young A was now 6 months past his fall and head injury. Although he was on medications, he continued to have intermittent seizures. The specialist adjusted his medications to better control these seizures. His disorder was diagnosed as _____

5. Baby Bobby was seen for his 6-month checkup. The physician checked his muscle tone and movement of all extremities. He also inquired about any sucking or feeding difficulties. This was part of the screening for a disorder that results from brain damage during the birth process, a condition known as _____

6. Ms. J, age 32, complained of weakness of the right side of the face, including drooping of the mouth and inability to close the right eye. The physician observed drooling from the right corner of the mouth and tears flowing from the right eye onto the cheek. A diagnosis of Bell's palsy was made. This disorder involves the cranial nerve named the _____

IX. Short Essays

1. Describe the structures that protect the brain and spinal cord.

_____

_____

_____

2. List some areas of the cerebral cortex that are involved in communication.

_____

_____

_____

3. List some functions of the structures in the diencephalon.

_____

_____

_____

11

The Sensory System

I. Overview

Through the functioning of the *sensory receptors*, we are made aware of changes taking place both internally and externally. Any change that produces a response in the nervous system is termed a *stimulus*.

The *special senses*, so called because the receptors are limited to a few specialized sense organs, include the senses of vision, hearing, equilibrium, taste, and smell. The receptors of the eye are the *rods* and *cones* located in the retina. The hearing receptors are found in a portion of the inner ear called the *cochlea*. Equilibrium receptors are in the vestibular apparatus of the inner ear. Receptors for the chemical senses of taste and smell are located on the tongue and in the upper part of the nose, respectively.

The *general senses* are scattered throughout the body; they respond to touch, pressure, temperature, pain, and position. Receptors for the sense of position, known as *proprioceptors*, are found in muscles, tendons, and joints.

The nerve impulses generated in a receptor cell by a stimulus must be carried to the central nervous system by way of a sensory (afferent) neuron. Here, the information is processed and a suitable response is made.

II. Topics for Review

A. The eye
  1. Protective structures of the eyeball
  2. Coats of the eyeball: sclera, choroid, retina
  3. Functions of the retina

III. Matching Exercises

Matching only within each group, write the answers in the spaces provided.

Group A

vitreous body   aqueous humor   choroid
accommodation   rods   cones
cornea   retina

1. The vascular, pigmented middle tunic of the eyeball   _____

2. The jellylike material located behind the crystalline lens that maintains the spherical shape of the eyeball   _____

3. The innermost coat of the eyeball, the nervous tissue layer that includes the receptors for the sense of vision   _____

4. The vision receptors that are sensitive to color   _____

5. The watery fluid that fills much of the eyeball in front of the crystalline lens   _____

6. The part of the eye that light rays pass through first as they enter the eye   _____

7. The process by which the lens becomes thicker to bend light rays for near vision   _____

8. The vision receptors that function in dim light   _____

Group B

conjunctiva   pupil   ciliary body
receptor   sclera   media
optic disk   iris

1. The colored part of the eye that regulates the size of the pupil   _____

2. The transparent refracting parts of the eye   _____

3. The muscle that alters the shape of the lens for accommodation   _____

4. The opaque outermost layer of the eyeball made of firm, tough connective tissue   _____

5. Another name for the blind spot, the region where the optic nerve connects with the eye   _____

6. The central opening in the iris   _____

7. The membrane that lines the eyelids _____

8. A part of the nervous system that detects a stimulus _____

Group C

rhodopsin	lacrimal gland	ophthalmia neonatorum
refraction	cataract	trachoma
extrinsic	intrinsic	fovea centralis

1. An opacity of the lens or its capsule _____

2. A serious eye infection of the newborn that can be prevented with a suitable antiseptic _____

3. Term that describes the muscles of the iris and ciliary body because they are located entirely within the eyeball _____

4. A structure that produces tears _____

5. The bending of light rays so that light from a large area can be focused on a small surface _____

6. A chronic eye infection for which antibiotics and proper hygiene have reduced the incidence of reinfection and blindness _____

7. Term for the muscles located outside the eyeball that are attached to bones of the orbit and to the sclera _____

8. The depressed area in the retina that is the point of clearest vision _____

9. A pigment needed for vision _____

Group D

strabismus	glaucoma	myopia
hyperopia	macular degeneration	crystalline lens
sphincter	astigmatism	

1. Eye disorder in which materials accumulate on the retina and gradually cause loss of vision _____

2. The scientific name for nearsightedness, in which the focal point is in front of the retina and distant objects appear blurred _____

3. The part of the eye that is removed in treatment of a cataract _____

4. The visual defect caused by irregularity in the curvature of the lens or cornea

_____

5. Condition in which the eyes do not work together because the muscles do not coordinate

_____

6. Condition caused by continued high pressure of the aqueous humor, which may result in destruction of the optic nerve fibers

_____

7. The scientific name for farsightedness, in which light rays are not bent sharply enough to focus on the retina when viewing close objects

_____

8. A circular muscle, such as the muscle of the iris

_____

Group E

oval window   mastoid air cells   tympanic membrane
ossicles   pinna   endolymph
perilymph   eustachian tube

1. The passageway that connects the middle ear cavity with the throat

_____

2. The fluid contained within the membranous labyrinth of the inner ear

_____

3. Another name for the projecting part, or auricle, of the ear

_____

4. The scientific name for the eardrum

_____

5. The membrane-covered space that conducts sound waves from the stapes to the fluid of the inner ear

_____

6. The spaces within the temporal bone that connect with the middle ear cavity through an opening

_____

7. The fluid of the inner ear contained within the bony labyrinth and surrounding the membranous labyrinth

_____

8. The three small bones within the middle ear cavity

_____

Group F

endorphin   vestibule   ophthalmic nerve
oculomotor nerve   cochlear duct   cochlear nerve
optic nerve   equilibrium

1. The entrance area that communicates with the cochlea and that is next to the oval window

_____

2. The branch of the fifth cranial nerve that carries impulses of pain, touch, and temperature from the eye to the brain

    _____

3. A pain reliever naturally released from the brain

    _____

4. The location of the organ of hearing

    _____

5. The largest of the three cranial nerves that carry motor fibers to the eyeball muscles

    _____

6. The sense that is located in the semicircular canals and the vestibule

    _____

7. The branch of the vestibulocochlear nerve that carries hearing impulses

    _____

8. The nerve that carries visual impulses from the retina to the brain

    _____

Group G

analgesic	proprioceptors	olfactory epithelium
glossopharyngeal	tactile corpuscles	ceruminous
adaptation	night blindness	

1. Receptors that transmit information on the position of body parts

    _____

2. One of the two nerves involved in the sense of taste

    _____

3. A drug that relieves pain

    _____

4. Term for the wax glands located in the external auditory canal

    _____

5. A condition that may result from a deficiency of vitamin A

    _____

6. Location of the receptors for the sense of smell

    _____

7. An adjustment to the environment so that one does not feel a sensation so acutely if a stimulus is continued

    _____

8. Receptors for the sense of touch

    _____

IV. Multiple Choice

Select the best answer and write the letter of your choice in the blank.

1. The term *lacrimation* refers to the secretion of

    1. _____

    a. mucus
    b. wax
    c. vitreous humor
    d. tears
    e. aqueous humor

2. A term related to the sense of taste is

    a. tactile
    b. aural
    c. gustatory
    d. proprioceptive
    e. thermal

2. _____

3. The nerves involved in the sense of taste are the

    a. vagus and vestibulocochlear
    b. oculomotor and trigeminal
    c. glossopharyngeal and olfactory
    d. ocular and abducens
    e. facial and glossopharyngeal

3. _____

4. A physician who specializes in disorders of the eye is a(n)

    a. ophthalmologist
    b. orthopedic surgeon
    c. internist
    d. allergist
    e. radiologist

4. _____

5. A cataract is

    a. an irregularity in the shape of the cornea
    b. loss of transparency of the lens
    c. an infection of the conjunctiva
    d. an abnormally short eyeball
    e. increased pressure in the eye

5. _____

6. A person who has a lack of cones in the retina will suffer from

    a. blindness
    b. color blindness
    c. presbyopia
    d. glaucoma
    e. trachoma

6. _____

7. The organ of Corti is the receptor for

    a. taste
    b. smell
    c. hearing
    d. pressure
    e. equilibrium

7. _____

8. Which of the following eye disorders does diabetes mellitus *not* contribute to?

    a. optic atrophy
    b. cataract
    c. retinal detachment
    d. enucleation
    e. retinopathy

8. _____

V. Labeling

For each of the following illustrations, write the name or names of each labeled part on the numbered lines.

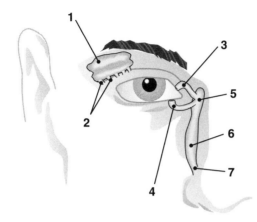

Lacrimal apparatus

1. _____

2. _____

3. _____

4. _____

5. _____

6. _____

7. _____

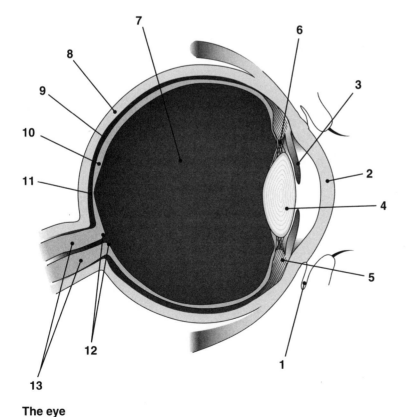

The eye

1. _____

2. _____

3. _____

4. _____

5. _____

6. _____

7. _____

8. _____

9. _____

10. _____

11. _____

12. _____

13. _____

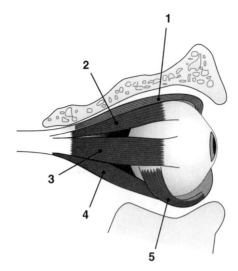

Extrinsic muscles of the eye

1. _____

2. _____

3. _____

4. _____

5. _____

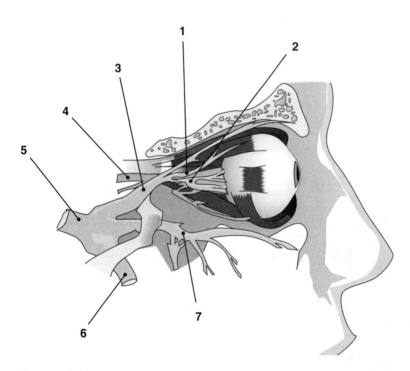

Nerves of the eye

1. _____   5. _____

2. _____   6. _____

3. _____   7. _____

4. _____

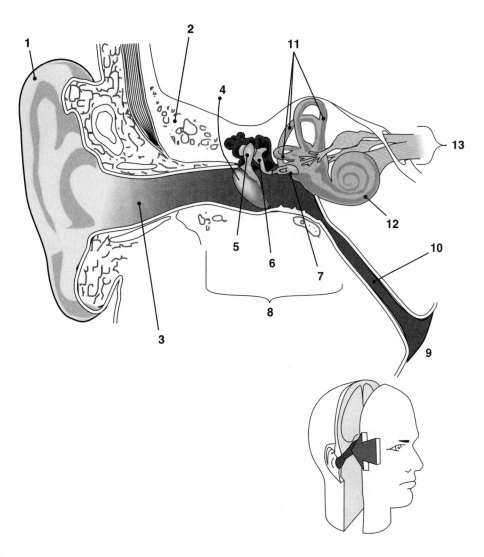

The ear

1. _____

2. _____

3. _____

4. _____

5. _____

6. _____

7. _____

8. _____

9. _____

10. _____

11. _____

12. _____

13. _____

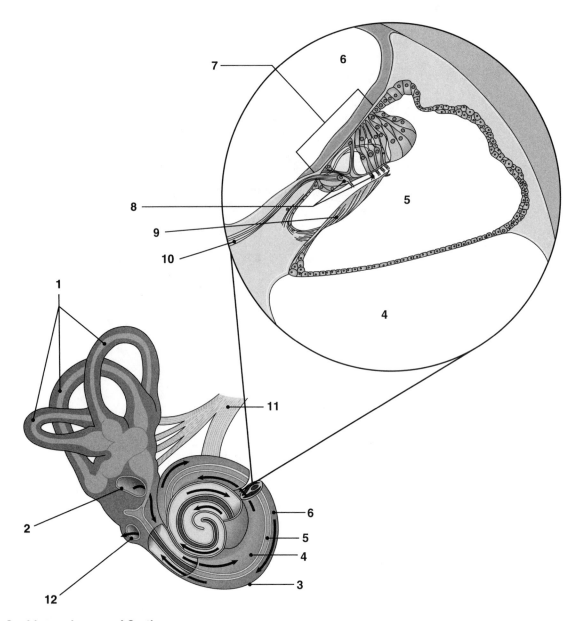

Cochlea and organ of Corti

1. _____

2. _____

3. _____

4. _____

5. _____

6. _____

7. _____

8. _____

9. _____

10. _____

11. _____

12. _____

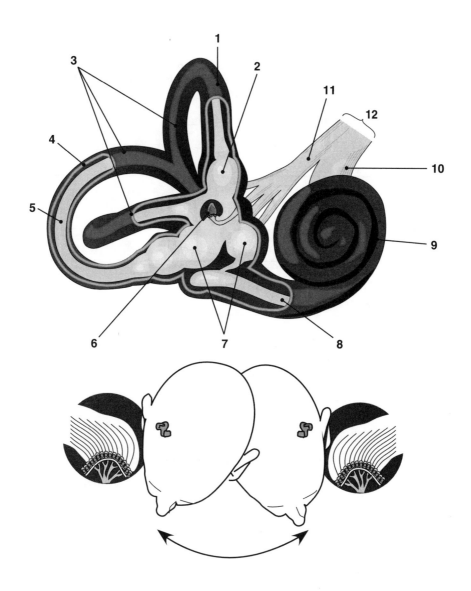

Inner ear

1. _____

2. _____

3. _____

4. _____

5. _____

6. _____

7. _____

8. _____

9. _____

10. _____

11. _____

12. _____

VI. True–False

For each question, write T for true or F for false in the blank to the left of each number. If a statement is false, correct it by replacing the underlined term and write the correct statement in the blanks below the question.

_____ 1. The middle coat, or tunic, of the eye is the sclera.

_____

_____

_____ 2. There are six extrinsic muscles connected to each eye.

_____

_____

_____ 3. The iris is an intrinsic muscle of the eye.

_____

_____

_____ 4. The sense of pressure is a special sense.

_____

_____

_____ 5. The rods of the eye function in bright light and detect color.

_____

_____

_____ 6. The scientific name for nearsightedness is hyperopia.

_____

_____

_____ 7. When the eyes are exposed to a bright light, the pupils contract.

_____

_____

_____ 8. Sound waves that enter the cochlea travel first through the tympanic duct.

_____

_____

_____ 9. The stapes is in contact with the oval window of the ear.

_____

_____

_____ 10. Perilymph is the fluid outside the membranous labyrinth of the ear.

_____

_____

_____ 11. The <u>aqueous humor</u> is the fluid in front of the lens of the eye.

_____

_____

_____ 12. Receptors for <u>static</u> equilibrium function when the body is spinning or moving in different directions.

_____

_____

VII. Completion Exercise

Write the word or phrase that correctly completes each sentence.

1. The bending of light rays as they pass through the media of the eye is   _____

2. The nerve fibers of the vestibular and cochlear nerves join to form the nerve called the   _____

3. The inner ear contains fluids involved in the transmission of sound waves. The fluid that is inside the membranous labyrinth of the cochlea is   _____

4. The very widely distributed free nerve endings are the receptors for the important protective sense of   _____

5. The tactile corpuscles are the receptors for the sense of   _____

6. The receptor tunic (layer) of the eye is the   _____

7. The nerve endings that aid in judging position and changes in location of body parts are the   _____

8. The sense of position is partially governed by several structures in the internal ear, including two small sacs in the vestibule and the three   _____

9. When you enter a darkened room, it takes a while for the rods to begin to function. This interval is known as the period of   _____

VIII. Practical Applications

Study each discussion. Then write the appropriate word or phrase in the space provided.

Group A

A student observed the following emergency cases seen by the eye specialist.

1. Ten-year-old K had been riding his bicycle and throwing glass bottles on the sidewalk. A fragment of glass flew into one eye. Examination by the eye specialist showed that there was a cut in the transparent window of the eye, the

   _____

2. On further examination of K, the colored part of the eye was seen to protrude from the wound. This part of the eye is the

   _____

3. K's treatment included antiseptics, anesthetics, and suturing of the wound. Medication was instilled in the saclike structure at the front of the eyeball. This sac is lined with a thin epithelial membrane, the

   _____

4. Mr. S, a construction worker, was brought in by his supervisor. He had been cutting metal without wearing his protective goggles, and a piece of steel had penetrated his eyeball. The physician found that jellylike material was protruding from the cut. This material, which maintains the shape of the eyeball, is the

   _____

5. Mr. W, a diabetic for 12 years, was referred due to sudden loss of vision in his left eye. The physician noted symptoms of diabetic retinopathy with evidence of a hemorrhage over the retina. The retina is the layer of the eye that contains the receptor cells known as

   _____

Group B

Dr. Garcia saw the following patients in her busy family practice clinic.

1. Mrs. B complained of some hearing loss and a sense of fullness in her outer ear. Examination revealed that her ear canal was plugged with hardened ear wax, which is scientifically called

   _____

2. Mr. J, age 72, complained of gradually increasing hearing loss, although he had no symptoms of pain or other problems related to the ears. Examination revealed that his hearing loss was due to nerve damage. The cranial nerve that carries hearing impulses to the brain is called the

   _____

3. Mrs. C complained of hearing loss that resembled the type from which her aunt and her mother suffered. She requested surgical treatment, which is often successful in such cases. This disorder, in which bony changes prevent the stapes from vibrating normally, is called

   _____

4. Baby L was brought in by his mother because he awakened crying and holding the right side of his head. He had been suffering from a cold, but now he seemed to be in pain. Examination revealed a bulging red eardrum. The eardrum is also called the

   _____

5. The cause of baby L's painful bulging eardrum was an infection of the middle ear, a condition called

_____

6. Antibiotic treatment of baby L's middle ear infection was begun, because this early treatment usually prevents complications. In this case, however, it was necessary to cut the eardrum to prevent its rupture. Another name for this surgical procedure is

_____

7. Elderly Mr. N had a hearing loss (presbycusis) due to atrophy of the nerve endings located in the spiral-shaped part of the inner ear, a part of the ear that is known as the

_____

8. Mr. N, age 86, had a weakness of the muscle that lifts the eyeball, the levator palpebrae. He complained of difficulty in seeing because of his drooping eyelids, a condition called

_____

IX. Short Essays

1. Describe several different forms of receptors and give examples of each.

_____

_____

_____

2. Compare the general and special senses and give examples of each.

_____

_____

_____

3. Define *sensory adaptation,* and cite its value.

_____

_____

_____

4. Describe some changes that occur in the sensory receptors with age.

_____

_____

_____

12

The Endocrine System: Glands and Hormones

I. Overview

Hormones are chemical messengers that have specific regulatory effects on certain other cells or organs in the body, the *target tissue.* Although hormones are produced by many tissues, hormone secretion is the primary function for certain glands. These are the *endocrine glands* or ductless glands, including the pituitary (hypophysis), thyroid, parathyroids, adrenals, pancreas, gonads, thymus, and pineal. Together, these comprise the *endocrine system.*

The endocrine system and the nervous system are the main coordinating and controlling systems of the body. Both are activated, for example, in helping the body respond to stress. These two systems meet in the *hypothalamus,* a region of the diencephalon of the brain. The hypothalamus, which is directly above and connected to the pituitary, governs both lobes of this gland. Hormones released from the pituitary, in turn, stimulate other endocrine glands. The main mechanism for controlling hormone secretion is *negative feedback,* in which hormone levels, or substances released as a result of hormone action, serve to regulate the production of that hormone.

Other structures that secrete hormones include the stomach, small intestine, kidney, heart, and placenta. *Prostaglandins* are hormones produced by cells throughout the body. They have a variety of effects and are currently under study.

II. Topics for Review

A. Hormones
1. Functions
2. Chemistry
3. Regulation

B. The endocrine glands and their hormones
   1. Control of the pituitary by the hypothalamus
C. Other hormone-producing organs
D. Hormones and treatment
E. Hormones and stress

III. Matching Exercises

Matching only within each group, write the answers in the spaces provided.

Group A

parathyroids	adrenal	hypothalamus
hormone	islets	thyroid
cretinism	pineal	

1. The largest of the endocrine glands, located in the neck

   _____

2. A substance produced by an endocrine gland

   _____

3. The endocrine gland composed of a cortex and medulla, each with specific functions

   _____

4. The tiny glands located behind the thyroid gland

   _____

5. The part of the brain that controls the pituitary gland

   _____

6. A condition that results from underactivity of the thyroid gland in infants and children   _____

7. The groups of hormone-secreting cells scattered throughout the pancreas   _____

8. The gland in the brain that is regulated by light   _____

Group B

pituitary   negative feedback   melatonin
suprarenal   calcitonin   target tissue
thyroxine   medulla

1. Another name for the adrenal gland   _____

2. The specific cells on which a hormone works   _____

3. The hormone produced by the thyroid gland that is active in calcium metabolism   _____

4. The self-regulating mechanism that controls hormone production   _____

5. The endocrine gland that is divided into an anterior and a posterior lobe   _____

6. The inner part of the adrenal gland   _____

7. The hormone produced by the pineal gland   _____

8. The hormone that is the main regulator of heat and energy production in the body   _____

Group C

adrenaline   insulin   parathyroid hormone
iodine   goiter   releasing hormone
myxedema   amino acid

1. Any enlargement of the thyroid gland   _____

2. A building block of protein hormones   _____

3. A hormone that lowers the level of sugar in the blood   _____

4. The chemical element that is needed for the manufacture of thyroxine   _____

5. A secretion that raises the level of calcium in the blood   _____

6. The common name for epinephrine   _____

7. A secretion from the hypothalamus that stimulates activity of the anterior lobe of the pituitary

_____

8. The condition caused by underactivity of the thyroid gland in the adult

_____

Group D

oxytocin   placenta   anterior lobe
thymosin   steroids   glucagon
cortisol   calcium

1. The chemical category that includes the sex hormones and the hormones of the adrenal cortex

_____

2. A hormone released by the adrenal cortex during stressful situations that acts to reduce inflammation

_____

3. The hormone that aids in maturation of the T cells needed for immunity

_____

4. The hormone produced by the pancreatic islets that raises blood sugar levels

_____

5. The part of the pituitary connected to the hypothalamus by a portal system

_____

6. The element regulated by hydroxycholecalciferol, a hormone produced from vitamin D

_____

7. An organ present only during pregnancy that secretes hormones needed for normal development of the embryo

_____

8. The hormone from the posterior pituitary that causes uterine contraction

_____

Group E

epinephrine   antidiuretic hormone   ACTH
luteinizing hormone   estrogen   kidney
aldosterone   somatotropin

1. The main hormone of the adrenal medulla that, among other actions, raises blood pressure and increases the heart rate

_____

2. The anterior pituitary hormone that stimulates the adrenal cortex

_____

3. A female sex hormone that most nearly parallels male testosterone in its action

_____

4. The hormone from the adrenal cortex that regulates the reabsorption of sodium and potassium in the kidney tubules

_____

5. The organ that produces erythropoietin, a hormone that stimulates production of red blood cells

_____

6. A gonadotropic hormone

_____

7. An alternate name for growth hormone

_____

8. The hormone produced in the posterior lobe of the pituitary that regulates water reabsorption by the kidney

_____

IV. Multiple Choice

Select the best answer and write the letter of your choice in the blank.

1. Another name for the pituitary gland is

   a. hypothalamus
   b. hypophysis
   c. thalamus
   d. cortex
   e. pineal

1. _____

2. Gonadotropins act on the

   a. kidneys and adrenal glands
   b. ovaries and testes
   c. hypothalamus and pituitary gland
   d. pineal body and thymus gland
   e. mammary glands and thyroid

2. _____

3. Which of the following hormones is *not* produced by the anterior pituitary?

   a. prolactin
   b. thyroid-stimulating hormone
   c. oxytocin
   d. luteinizing hormone
   e. growth hormone

3. _____

4. An excess of growth hormone in an adult results in

   a. acromegaly
   b. diabetes insipidus
   c. tetany
   d. myxedema
   e. goiter

4. _____

5. An androgen is a(n)

   a. female sex hormone
   b. glucocorticoid
   c. lymphocyte
   d. male sex hormone
   e. atrial hormone

5. _____

6. Diabetes insipidus results from a deficiency of

   a. ACTH
   b. thymosin
   c. ADH
   d. melatonin
   e. ICSH

6. _____

7. Addison's disease results from underactivity of the

   a. ovary
   b. adrenal medulla
   c. anterior pituitary
   d. parathyroid
   e. adrenal cortex

7. _____

8. The gland active in immunity is the

   a. thyroid
   b. thymus
   c. pineal
   d. kidney
   e. posterior pituitary

8. _____

V. Labeling

For each of the following illustrations, write the name or names of each labeled part on the numbered lines.

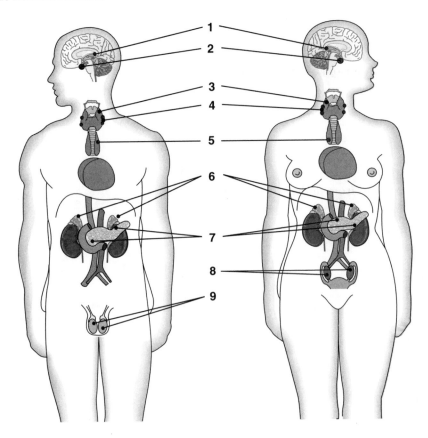

The endocrine glands

1. _____

2. _____

3. _____

4. _____

5. _____

6. _____

7. _____

8. _____

9. _____

Thyroid gland

1. _____

2. _____

3. _____

4. _____

5. _____

6. _____

7. _____

VI. True–False

For each question, write T for true or F for false in the blank to the left of each number. If a statement is false, correct it by replacing the underlined term and write the correct statement in the blanks below the question.

_____ 1. The ovaries and testes produce <u>steroid</u> hormones.

_____

_____

_____ 2. Islet cells are found in the <u>adrenal</u> gland.

_____

_____

_____ 3. ADH and oxytocin are secreted by the <u>anterior</u> lobe of the pituitary.

_____

_____

_____ 4. <u>Glucagon</u> is the pancreatic hormone that lowers blood sugar levels.

_____

_____

_____ 5. Parathyroid hormone <u>raises</u> calcium levels in the blood.

_____

_____

_____ 6. Graves' disease is caused by an overactive <u>thyroid</u> gland.

_____

_____

_____ 7. <u>IDDM</u> is the form of diabetes mellitus that usually appears at a young age.

_____

_____

_____ 8. Atrial natriuretic peptide (ANP) is produced by the <u>kidneys</u>.

_____

_____

VII. Completion Exercise

Write the word or phrase that correctly completes each sentence.

1. The region of the brain that controls the pituitary
   gland is the   _____

2. If the production of parathyroid hormone decreases below
   normal levels, there is a decrease in the amount of calcium
   dissolved in the blood. This may be followed by muscle
   spasms, a condition called   _____

3. An abnormal increase in production of the hormone
   epinephrine may result from a tumor of the   _____

4. The immune system is stimulated by the hormone from
   the thymus gland called   _____

5. Releasing hormones are sent from the hypothalamus to
   the anterior pituitary by way of a special circulatory
   pathway called a(n)   _____

6. The hypothalamus stimulates the anterior pituitary to produce
   ACTH, which, in turn, stimulates hormone production by the _____

7. Local hormones that have a variety of effects, including the promotion of inflammation and the production of uterine contractions, are the

_____

8. When the level of glucose in the blood decreases to less than average, the islet cells of the pancreas release less insulin. The result is an increase in blood glucose. This is an example of the regulatory mechanism called

_____

VIII. Practical Applications

Study each discussion. Then write the appropriate word or phrase in the space provided.

1. Mr. J, age 52, required evaluation of pituitary function. He showed abnormal weakness, enlargement of his hands and feet, and facial changes. Imaging studies and other tests revealed that a pituitary tumor was causing excess production of growth hormone. His condition was diagnosed as

_____

2. Seventeen-year-old Ms. K had never had a menstrual period. The cause was diagnosed as a deficiency of the ovarian hormones called   ·

_____

3. Mrs. C, age 56, although she had fatigue and unexplained weight loss for several months, was just now reporting to the physician. A blood chemistry panel taken when she had not eaten for 8 hours showed a blood glucose reading of 186 mg/dL as well as other abnormal readings. A disorder of insulin production was suspected, leading to a tentative diagnosis of

_____

4. Mrs. K was brought in by her husband, who was concerned about her weakness and weight loss. The physician noted muscle wasting and bronze skin. Laboratory tests showed a deficiency in cortisol as well as abnormal electrolytes. On this basis, the physician made a diagnosis of hypofunction of the adrenal cortex, a disorder known as

_____

5. Mr. L, age 42, reported to the hospital emergency room with complaints of shortness of breath and heart palpitation. The initial assessment by the nurse included the following findings: rapid heart rate, nervousness with tremor of the hands, skin warm and flushed, sweating, rapid respiration, and protruding eyes. Laboratory tests confirmed the diagnosis of overactivity of the

_____

6. After surgery for his endocrine problem, Mr. L had tetany, or contractions of the muscles of the hands and face. This was caused by the incidental surgical removal of the glands that control the release of calcium into the blood. The glands that maintain adequate blood calcium levels are the _____

7. Mr. G, age 38, had been taking high doses of oral steroid drugs for asthma for 6 years. He noted fat deposits between his shoulders and around his abdomen, muscle loss in his arms and legs, and thin skin that was prone to bruising. The doctor ordered a test of bone density and a blood chemistry test. These symptoms are common with excess of hormones produced normally by the _____

IX. Short Essays

1. Describe the characteristics of hormones.

   _____

   _____

   _____

2. Explain why hormones, although they circulate throughout the body, exercise their effects only on specific target cells.

   _____

   _____

   _____

3. Compare the anterior and the posterior lobes of the pituitary.

   _____

   _____

   _____

4. Some endocrine glands produce hormones, known as *tropic hormones,* that stimulate other endocrine glands. Name several such tropic hormones and explain what each does.

_____

_____

_____

Unit V

CIRCULATION AND BODY DEFENSE

13

The Blood

I. Overview

The blood maintains the constancy of the internal environment through its functions of transportation, regulation, and protection. Blood is composed of two elements: the liquid element, or *plasma,* and the *formed elements,* consisting of the cells and cellular products. The plasma is 90% water and 10% proteins, carbohydrates, lipids, electrolytes, and waste products. The formed elements are composed of the *erythrocytes,* which carry oxygen to the tissues; the *leukocytes,* which defend the body against invaders; and the *platelets,* which are involved in the process of blood coagulation (clotting). The forerunners of the blood cells are called *stem cells.* These are formed in the red bone marrow, where they then develop into the various types of blood cells.

Blood *coagulation* is a protective mechanism that prevents blood loss when a blood vessel is ruptured by an injury. The steps in the prevention of blood loss (hemostasis) include constriction of the blood vessels, formation of a platelet plug, and formation of a clot, a complex series of reactions involving 12 different factors.

If the quantity of blood in the body is severely reduced because of hemorrhage or disease, the cells suffer from lack of oxygen and nutrients. In such instances, a *transfusion* may be given after typing and matching the blood of the donor with that of the recipient. Donor red cells with different surface *antigens* (proteins) than the recipient's red cells will react with *antibodies* in the recipient's blood, causing harmful agglutination reactions and destruction of the donated cells. Blood is most commonly tested for the ABO system involving antigens A and B. Blood can be packaged and stored in blood banks for use when transfusions are needed. Whenever possible, *blood components* such as cells, plasma,

plasma fractions, or platelets are used. This practice is more efficient and can reduce the chances of incompatibility and transmission of disease.

The *Rh factor,* another red blood cell protein, also is important in transfusions. If blood containing the Rh factor (Rh positive) is given to a person whose blood lacks that factor (Rh negative), the recipient will produce antibodies to the foreign Rh factor. If an Rh-negative mother is thus sensitized by an Rh-positive fetus, her antibodies may damage fetal red cells in a later pregnancy, resulting in *hemolytic disease of the newborn* (erythroblastosis fetalis).

Anemia is a common blood disorder. It may result from loss or destruction of red blood cells or from impaired production of red blood cells or hemoglobin. Other abnormalities are *leukemia,* a neoplastic disease of white cells, and *clotting disorders.*

Numerous *blood studies* have been devised to measure the composition of blood. These include the hematocrit, hemoglobin measurements, cell counts, blood chemistry tests, and coagulation studies. Modern laboratories are equipped with automated counters, which rapidly and accurately count blood cells, and with automated analyzers, which measure enzymes, electrolytes, and other constituents of blood serum.

II. Topics for Review

A. Functions of blood
B. Blood plasma and its functions
C. The formed elements and their functions
    1. Erythrocytes
        a. Structure
        b. Function

         2. Leukocytes
            a. Types
            b. Functions
         3. Platelets (thrombocytes)
      D. Origin of the formed elements
      E. Hemostasis
         1. Blood clotting
      F. Blood types
         1. ABO
         2. Rh
      G. Uses of blood and blood components
         1. Blood banks
         2. Transfusions
      H. Blood disorders
      I. Blood studies

III. Matching Exercises

Matching only within each group, write the answers in the spaces provided.

Group A

erythrocyte	thrombocyte	carbon dioxide
oxygen	plasma	red marrow
hemoglobin	leukocyte	

1. A white blood cell   _____

2. The connective tissue in bone that is the site of blood
   cell formation   _____

3. The liquid part of the blood   _____

4. The gaseous waste product carried by the blood to the lungs _____

5. A red blood cell   _____

6. The important gas that is transported by the blood from
   the lungs to all parts of the body   _____

7. Another name for a platelet, an element active in
   blood clotting   _____

8. The pigment in red blood cells that carries oxygen   _____

Group B

gamma globulin	cryoprecipitate	plasmapheresis
hemostasis	albumin	antigens
neutrophils	Rh	sickle cell anemia

1. The proteins on the surface of the red blood cells that limit
   the types of transfusions that can be given to a person   _____

2. A blood fraction obtained from frozen plasma that contains clotting factors

_____

3. The fraction of the blood that contains antibodies

_____

4. A hereditary hemolytic disease seen mainly in blacks

_____

5. The procedure for removing plasma and returning formed elements to a donor

_____

6. The most numerous leukocytes in the blood

_____

7. The blood antigen involved in hemolytic disease of the newborn, which results from a blood incompatibility between a mother and a fetus

_____

8. The most abundant protein in the blood

_____

9. The name for the process that prevents blood loss

_____

Group C

stem cells	agglutination	megakaryocytes
hemolysis	hemoglobin	pus
fibrinogen	serum	

1. A substance that often accumulates when leukocytes are actively destroying bacteria

_____

2. The watery fluid that remains after a clot is removed

_____

3. The substance in red blood cells that contains iron

_____

4. A plasma protein that is activated to form a blood clot

_____

5. The process by which cells become clumped when mixed with a specific antiserum

_____

6. The rupture of red blood cells

_____

7. The ancestors of all blood cells

_____

8. The large cells that give off fragments known as platelets

_____

Group D

purpura	anemia	hemorrhage
centrifuge	transfusion	vitamin B_{12}
electrolytes	leukemia	

1. The substance needed for red cell formation, the lack of which will result in pernicious anemia

_____

2. A neoplastic disease in which there is an abnormal increase in the number of immature white cells

_____

3. The salts that are dissolved in body fluids such as plasma

_____

4. The condition in which the blood is lacking in red blood cells or hemoglobin

_____

5. A machine that is used to separate the blood cells from blood plasma

_____

6. Another term for profuse abnormal bleeding

_____

7. The administration of blood or blood components from one person to another person

_____

8. A disorder in which there are hemorrhages into the skin and mucous membranes

_____

Group E

hemocytometer	leukocytosis	4.5 to 5 million
leukopenia	hyperglycemia	hematocrit
5,000 to 10,000		

1. The test that measures the volume percentage of red blood cells in centrifuged whole blood

_____

2. The average number of white cells per cubic millimeter of blood

_____

3. An apparatus used for manual counts of blood cells

_____

4. The average number of red cells per cubic millimeter of blood

_____

5. An excessive white blood cell count, as seen in cases of infection

_____

6. An excessive amount of sugar in the blood, as seen in unregulated diabetes

_____

7. A reduction of the white cell count to below the normal range

_____

IV. Multiple Choice

Select the best answer and write the letter of your choice in the blank.

1. Carbon monoxide can block the ability of the blood to carry

1. _____

   a. carbon dioxide
   b. oxygen
   c. hemoglobin
   d. albumin
   e. plasma

2. Next to water, the most abundant material in blood plasma is

    a. urea
    b. glucose
    c. protein
    d. vitamins
    e. carbon dioxide

2. _____

3. Which of the following is *not* a function of blood?

    a. transportation of waste products
    b. transportation of nutrients
    c. distribution of heat
    d. hemostasis
    e. manufacture of hormones

3. _____

4. Polymorphs, PMNs, and segs are alternate names for

    a. neutrophils
    b. basophils
    c. lymphocytes
    d. eosinophils
    e. monocytes

4. _____

5. Which of the following is *not* a type of white blood cell?

    a. thrombocyte
    b. eosinophil
    c. neutrophil
    d. monocyte
    e. lymphocyte

5. _____

6. Autologous blood is

    a. blood that has been frozen
    b. blood that has been typed
    c. incompatible blood
    d. a person's own blood
    e. blood that has been separated

6. _____

7. Blood clotting occurs in a complex series of steps. The substance that finally forms the clot is

    a. anticoagulant
    b. thromboplastin
    c. antibody
    d. fibrin
    e. albumin

7. _____

8. Which of the following might result in an Rh incompatibility problem?

    a. an Rh-positive mother and an Rh-negative fetus
    b. an Rh-negative mother and an Rh-positive fetus
    c. an Rh-negative mother and a type AB fetus
    d. an Rh-positive mother and an Rh-negative father
    e. an Rh-positive mother and an Rh-positive father

8. _____

9. Plasma can be given to anyone without danger of incompatibility because it lacks

9. _____

   a. serum
   b. thrombocytes
   c. red cells
   d. protein
   e. clotting factors

10. Intrinsic factor is

10. _____

   a. the first factor activated in blood clotting
   b. a substance needed for absorption of folic acid
   c. a cause of leukemia
   d. a substance needed for absorption of vitamin B_{12}
   e. a type of hereditary bleeding disease

V. Labeling

For each of the following illustrations, write the name or names of each labeled part on the numbered lines.

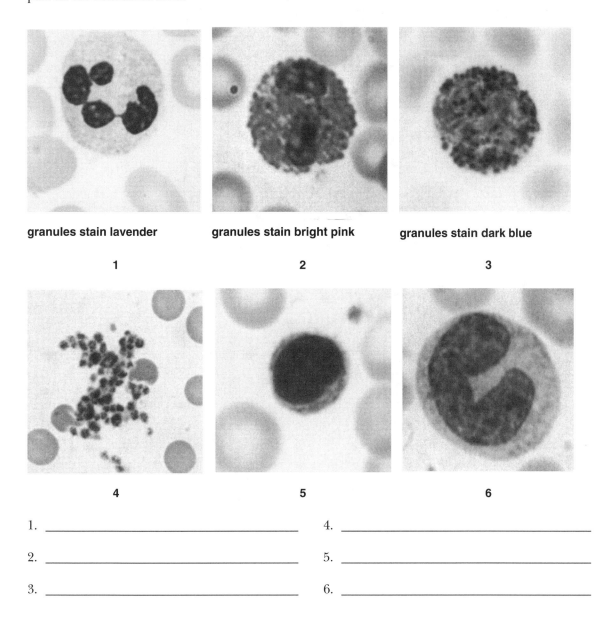

granules stain lavender   granules stain bright pink   granules stain dark blue

1   2   3

4   5   6

1. _____   4. _____

2. _____   5. _____

3. _____   6. _____

Anti-A serum   **Anti-B serum**

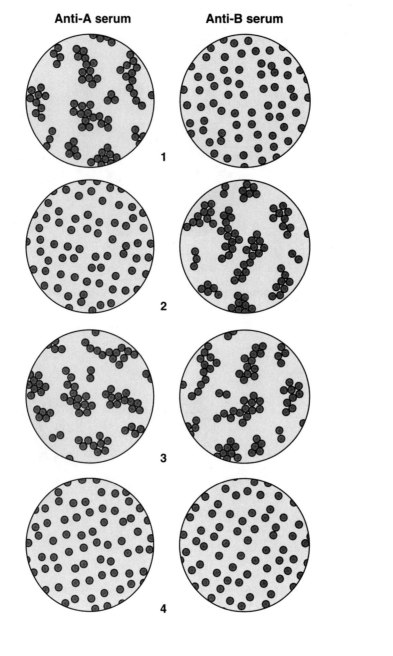

1

2

3

4

Blood typing

1. _____   3. _____

2. _____   4. _____

VI. True–False

For each question, write T for true or F for false in the blank to the left of each number. If a statement is false, correct it by replacing the underlined term and write the correct statement in the blanks below the question.

_____ 1. Blood from a person with type A blood will agglutinate with type B antiserum.

_____

_____

_____ 2. Type O blood contains antibodies to both A and B antigens.

_____

_____

_____ 3. Lymphocytes and monocytes are granular leukocytes.

_____

_____

_____ 4. The form of leukemia that arises in bone marrow is myelogenous leukemia.

_____

_____

_____ 5. Erythropoietin, a hormone that stimulates production of red blood cells, is produced by the kidneys.

_____

_____

_____ 6. Band cells are immature neutrophils.

_____

_____

_____ 7. Substances that prevent blood clotting are called procoagulants.

_____

_____

_____ 8. The watery fluid that remains after a blood clot has been removed from the blood is <u>plasma</u>.

_____

_____

VII. Completion Exercise

Write the word or phrase that correctly completes each sentence.

1. The gas that is necessary for life and that is transported to all parts of the body by the blood is _____

2. One waste product of body metabolism is carried to the lungs to be exhaled. This gas is _____

3. Blood cells are formed in the _____

4. The liquid fraction of the blood is _____

5. The number of different types of granular white blood cells is _____

6. Some monocytes enter the tissues, mature, and become active phagocytes. These cells are called _____

7. The process whereby red blood cells are clumped together in a reaction with a specific antiserum is _____

8. The most important function of certain lymphocytes is to engulf disease-producing organisms by the process of _____

9. The chemical element that characterizes hemoglobin is _____

VIII. Practical Applications

Study each discussion. Then write the appropriate word or phrase in the space provided.

Group A

1. Teenage RG sustained numerous deep gashes when he reached through a store window that he and his friends had broken. One of the cuts bled copiously. In describing this type of bleeding, the doctor in the emergency clinic used the word _____

2. While the physician attended to the wound, the technician drew blood for typing and other studies. RG's blood was found to agglutinate with both anti-A and anti-B serum. His blood was classified as group

_____

3. Among the available donors were some whose blood was found to be free of both A and B surface antigens. They were classified as having blood type

_____

4. Further testing of RG's blood revealed that it lacked the Rh factor. He was, therefore, said to be

_____

5. If RG were to be given a transfusion of Rh-positive blood, he might become sensitized to the Rh protein. In that event, his blood would produce counteracting substances called

_____

Group B

1. Mr. B had a history of peptic ulcer. Earlier, he had passed a black stool. Now, he was dizzy. He reported to the emergency clinic where they tested his hemoglobin level and hematocrit. The results showed a serious decrease in both measures of red cells. The name of this condition, for which there are many causes is

_____

2. Mr. R had lost a large quantity of blood when he was injured in an automobile accident. In addition to whole blood, he was given several units of cryoprecipitate to replace lost

_____

3. Mr. J, a kidney transplant patient, reported to his physician's office. He was maintained on drugs to suppress the immune system and was going to visit a foreign country where hepatitis is common. For his protection, he was to be given an injection of plasma containing antibodies. The fraction of the plasma that contains antibodies is

_____

4. Teenage Joyce visited the prenatal clinic. She was noted to be listless and pale. Her diet consisted largely of fast foods and snack items. Her condition was due to dietary deficiency of iron and vitamins, which resulted in a form of anemia known as

_____

5. Lester, age 9, had played a long, hard game of hockey one cool November day. Later, his mother brought him to the hospital emergency department with severe pain and swelling of the hands and feet. Lester was diagnosed as having painful crisis. He was known to have a disorder of hemoglobin that causes RBCs to assume an abnormal shape. The name of this condition is

_____

Group C

The medical laboratory that processed specimens for the hospital and a nearby medical office building had test orders for clients with the following histories.

1. A 5-year-old boy had a history of frequent fevers and a tendency to bleed easily. His skin was pale and his heart rate rapid. The laboratory estimated the percentage of the different types of white cells in a blood smear, a test called a(n) _____

2. Further study of this patient's blood smear revealed that numerous white blood cells were immature, and that the total number of white cells was tremendously increased. This disorder, a cancer of the blood, is _____

3. As a further aid in diagnosis, a specimen of his red marrow was obtained from the iliac crest by means of a special needle. This procedure is a(n) _____

4. Mrs. C's history included rapid weight loss, constant thirst, and episodes of fainting. Tests showed the presence of excessive sugar, or glucose, in the blood. This symptom is described as _____

5. Mr. B, age 28, had a history of heart disease due to bacteria that caused dissolution (dissolving) of red blood cells. This disintegration of red blood cells is known as _____

IX. Short Essays

1. What precautions must be taken when whole blood is transfused from one person to another?

   _____

   _____

   _____

2. What is anemia, and what are some possible causes of anemia?

   _____

   _____

   _____

3. What kind of information can be obtained from blood chemistry tests?

_____

_____

_____

14

The Heart and Heart Disease

I. Overview

The ceaseless beat of the heart day and night throughout one's entire lifetime is such an obvious key to the presence of life that it is no surprise that this organ has been the subject of wonderment and poetry. When the heart stops pumping, life ceases. The cells must have oxygen, and it is the heart's pumping action that propels oxygenated blood to them.

In size, the heart is roughly the size of one's fist. It is located between the lungs, more than half to the left of the midline, with the *apex* (point) directed toward the left. Below is the *diaphragm,* the dome-shaped muscle that separates the thoracic cavity from the abdominopelvic cavity.

The heart has two sides, in which blood that is higher in oxygen is kept entirely separate from blood that is lower in oxygen. The two sides pump in unison, the right side pumping blood to the lungs to be oxygenated, and the left side pumping blood to all other parts of the body.

Each side of the heart is divided into two parts or *chambers,* which are in direct communication. The upper chamber or *atrium* on each side is the receiving chamber for blood returning to the heart. The lower chamber or *ventricle* is the strong pumping chamber. Because the ventricles pump more forcefully, their walls are thicker than the walls of the atria. *Valves* between the chambers keep the blood flowing forward as the heart pumps. The muscle of the heart wall, the *myocardium,* has special features to enhance its pumping efficiency. The coronary circulation supplies blood directly to the myocardium.

The heartbeat originates within the heart at the *sinoatrial (SA) node,* often called the pacemaker. Electrical impulses from the pacemaker spread over special fibers in the wall of the heart to produce contractions, first of the two atria and then of the two ventricles. After contraction, the heart relaxes and fills with blood. The relaxation phase is called *diastole,* and the contraction phase is called *systole.* Together, these two phases make up one *cardiac cycle.* The heart rate is influenced by the nervous system and other circulating factors, such as hormones and drugs.

Heart diseases may be classified according to the area of the heart affected or according to causes. Causes include congenital abnormalities, rheumatic fever, coronary artery disease, and heart failure.

II. Topics for Review

A. Structure of the heart wall
   1. Endocardium
   2. Myocardium
   3. Epicardium
      a. Pericardium
B. Structure of the heart
   1. Septum
   2. Chambers
   3. Valves
C. Work of the heart
   1. Blood circuits
      a. Pulmonary
      b. Systemic
   2. The cardiac cycle
      a. Diastole
      b. Systole
   3. Cardiac output

4. The conduction system of the heart
   a. Sinoatrial node (pacemaker)
   b. Atrioventricular node
   c. Atrioventricular bundle and bundle branches
   d. Purkinje fibers
5. Heart rate
6. Normal and abnormal sounds
D. Heart disease
   1. Classification
   2. Descriptions
   3. The heart in the elderly
   4. Prevention of heart ailments
   5. Instruments used in diagnosis
   6. Treatment
      a. Drugs
      b. Pacemakers
      c. Surgery

III. Matching Exercises

Matching only within each group, write the answers in the spaces provided.

Group A

ventricles	tricuspid valve	aortic valve
endocardium	myocardium	pulmonic valve
mitral valve	epicardium	atria

1. The left atrioventricular valve _____

2. The heart muscle, the thickest layer in the heart wall _____

3. The lower chambers of the heart _____

4. The valve that prevents blood on its way to the lungs from returning to the right ventricle _____

5. The membrane that forms the heart valves and lines the interior of the heart _____

6. The outermost layer of the heart _____

7. The upper chambers of the heart _____

8. The valve that prevents blood from returning to the left ventricle _____

9. The right atrioventricular valve _____

Group B

arteries	sinoatrial node	systole
interventricular septum	veins	diastole
atrioventricular node	atrioventricular bundle	interatrial septum

1. The group of conduction fibers between the AV node and the ventricles

_____

2. The partition between the two lower chambers of the heart

_____

3. The contraction phase of the cardiac cycle

_____

4. Vessels that carry blood from the tissues back to the heart

_____

5. The resting period that follows the contraction phase of the cardiac cycle

_____

6. The pacemaker of the heart, located in the upper wall of the right atrium

_____

7. The mass of conduction tissue located in the septum at the bottom of the right atrium

_____

8. Vessels that carry blood from the heart to the tissues

_____

9. The partition that separates the two upper chambers of the heart

_____

Group C

atherosclerosis	tachycardia	bicuspid
murmur	flutter	cardiac output
myocardium	bradycardia	stroke volume

1. Alternate name for the mitral valve

_____

2. Term for a heart rate of greater than 100 beats per minute

_____

3. The tissue that is supplied by the coronary arteries

_____

4. Term for very rapid coordinated heart contractions of up to 300 beats per minute

_____

5. A sound that may result from a heart defect, such as the abnormal closing of a heart valve

_____

6. The amount of blood ejected from a ventricle with each beat

_____

7. A heart rate of less than 60 beats per minute

_____

8. Degenerative process that gradually produces thickening and hardening of vessels

_____

9. The volume of blood pumped by each ventricle in 1 minute

_____

Group D

fibrillation	thrombus	functional
endocarditis	congenital	ischemia
myocarditis	occlusion	infarct

1. Inflammation of the heart lining, often affecting the valves _____

2. A blood clot formed within a blood vessel _____

3. A general term that is used to describe heart abnormalities and other defects that have been present since birth _____

4. Condition that results from a lack of blood supply to the tissues, as from narrowing of an artery _____

5. Inflammation of heart muscle _____

6. Rapid, wild, uncoordinated contractions of the heart muscle _____

7. Term used for the type of murmur that is associated with normal function of the heart _____

8. Complete closure, as of an artery _____

9. An area of dead tissue damaged by a lack of blood supply _____

Group E

catheterization	digitalis	anticoagulant
coronary thrombosis	cyanosis	electrocardiograph
artificial pacemaker	hypertension	stethoscope

1. The medical term for high blood pressure _____

2. A drug that may be prescribed to prevent the formation of a thrombus in a blood vessel _____

3. A simple instrument used by medical personnel for listening to sounds from within the patient's body _____

4. Blueness of the skin caused by lack of oxygen supply _____

5. A device implanted under the skin that supplies impulses to regulate the heartbeat _____

6. A procedure for measuring pressures within the heart chambers and checking the function of the heart valves _____

7. Formation of a blood clot within an artery of the heart, thus obstructing blood flow _____

8. A valuable drug derived from the foxglove plant that aids in regulating the heartbeat _____

9. An instrument for recording the electrical activity of the heart _____

IV. Multiple Choice

Select the best answer and write the letter of your choice in the blank.

1. The special membranes between cardiac muscle cells are called

   a. interfaces
   b. intercalated disks
   c. chordae tendineae
   d. foramen ovale
   e. coarctations

   1. _____

2. An average cardiac cycle lasts about

   a. 8 seconds
   b. 5 seconds
   c. 1 minute
   d. 0.8 second
   e. 30 seconds

   2. _____

3. Discomfort felt in the region of the heart as a result of coronary artery disease is called

   a. fibrillation
   b. heart block
   c. angina pectoris
   d. hypertension
   e. extrasystole

   3. _____

4. The circulatory system of the fetus has certain adaptations for the purpose of bypassing the

   a. heart
   b. lungs
   c. placenta
   d. kidneys
   e. umbilical cord

   4. _____

5. Which of the following is *not* a part of the conduction system of the heart?

   a. bundle of His
   b. right bundle branch
   c. Purkinje fibers
   d. calcium channel
   e. atrioventricular node

   5. _____

6. The vein that carries blood from the coronary circulation back into the right atrium is the

   a. right coronary artery
   b. epicardium
   c. interatrial septum
   d. heart block
   e. coronary sinus

   6. _____

7. The function of a thrombolytic drug is to

   a. dissolve blood clots
   b. reduce hypertension
   c. regulate the heartbeat
   d. dilate the blood vessels
   e. reduce the force of heart contractions

7. _____

8. An autonomic nerve that directly affects the heart rate is the

   a. vagus
   b. accessory
   c. oculomotor
   d. glossopharyngeal
   e. trigeminal

8. _____

V. Labeling

For each of the following illustrations, write the name or names of each labeled part on the numbered lines.

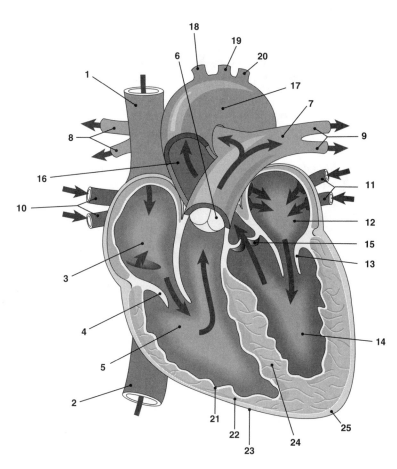

Heart and great vessels

1. _____

2. _____

3. _____

4. _____

5. _____

6. _____

7. _____

8. _____

9. _____

10. _____

11. _____

12. _____

13. _____

14. _____

15. _____

16. _____

17. _____

18. _____

19. _____

20. _____

21. _____

22. _____

23. _____

24. _____

25. _____

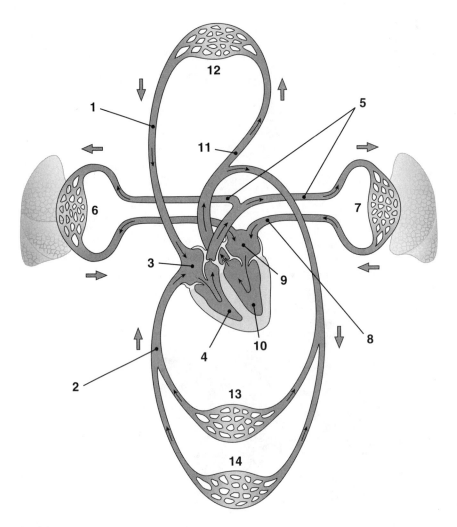

The heart is a double pump

1. _____

2. _____

3. _____

4. _____

5. _____

6. _____

7. _____

8. _____

9. _____

10. _____

11. _____

12. _____

13. _____

14. _____

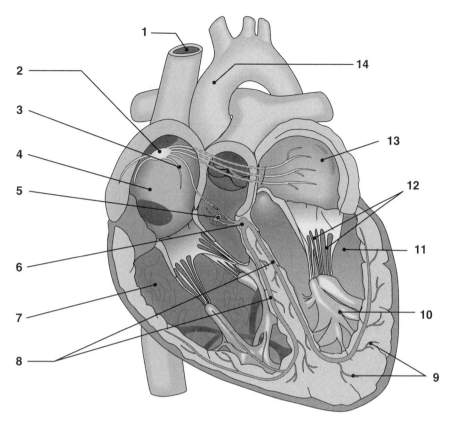

Conduction system of the heart

1. _____

2. _____

3. _____

4. _____

5. _____

6. _____

7. _____

8. _____

9. _____

10. _____

11. _____

12. _____

13. _____

14. _____

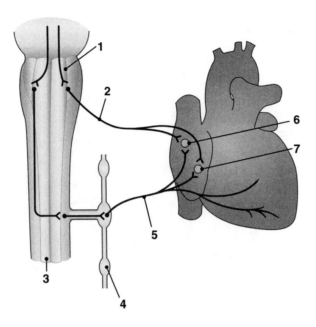

Nervous stimulation of the heart

1. _____   5. _____

2. _____   6. _____

3. _____   7. _____

4. _____

VI. True–False

For each question, write T for true or F for false in the blank to the left of each number. If a statement is false, correct it by replacing the underlined term and write the correct statement in the blanks below the question.

_____ 1. The right atrioventricular valve is the <u>bicuspid</u> valve.

_____

_____

_____ 2. The <u>systemic</u> circuit carries blood to the lungs.

_____

_____

_____ 3. The <u>epicardium</u> is the tissue that lines the interior of the heart.

_____

_____

_____ 4. A normal heart rhythm, or sinus rhythm, originates at the <u>sinoatrial</u> node.

_____

_____

_____ 5. When the ventricles contract, the atrioventricular valves are <u>closed.</u>

_____

_____

_____ 6. A rapid heart rate is described as <u>bradycardia.</u>

_____

_____

_____ 7. Stimulation from the sympathetic nervous system <u>increases</u> the heart rate.

_____

_____

_____ 8. The vagus nerve is part of the <u>sympathetic</u> nervous system.

_____

_____

VII. Completion Exercise

Write the word or phrase that correctly completes each sentence.

1. The fibrous sac that surrounds the heart is the _____

2. A partition between chambers of the heart is a(n) _____

3. Because each flap of the aortic and pulmonary valves is halfmoon-shaped, these valves are described as _____

4. Another name for the left atrioventricular valve is the _____

5. One complete sequence of relaxation and contraction of the heart is called a(n) _____

6. The stroke volume and heart rate determine the volume of blood pumped by each ventricle in 1 minute. This volume is termed the _____

7. The main influence over the heart rate outside of the heart itself is the _____

8. A rapid, painless, and harmless method for studying the heart uses sound impulses that are reflected and recorded. This method is named _____

9. An abnormality in the rhythm of the heartbeat is termed _____

10. A device used to restore a normal heart rhythm by stimulating cardiac muscle cells with a strong electrical current is a(n) _____

VIII. Practical Applications

Study each discussion. Then write the appropriate word or phrase in the space provided.

Group A

1. Mrs. K had rheumatic fever several times during her teenage years. Now, in middle age, she is often short of breath and complains of spitting up blood. It is found that her left atrio-ventricular valve has become so scarred that blood cannot flow adequately from the left atrium to the left ventricle. Scarring of the mitral valve so that it does not open sufficiently is called _____

2. Using the stethoscope to listen to Mrs. K's heart, the physician detected an abnormal sound termed a(n) _____

3. Mrs. K underwent a procedure during which a small tube was introduced into the veins of her right arm and then into the right side of the heart. This procedure is called _____

4. Mr. L was 42 years of age and overweight. During a game of handball, he felt severe heart pains and collapsed in shock. Testing indicated that a clot had formed in a blood vessel supplying an area of heart muscle resulting in complete obstruction of blood flow. Formation of a blood clot in a heart vessel is called _____

5. Mr. S, age 72, came to the physician's office complaining of shortness of breath. It was noted that his weight had increased 12 lb since his last visit. There was evidence of fluid retention in the lower extremities and abdomen as well as abnormal breath sounds. A chest x-ray study revealed an enlarged heart indicating a disorder called _____

Group B

1. Mr. B, age 54, was shopping in the mall when he suddenly collapsed with chest pain. The paramedics were preparing him for transport to the hospital when they noted a sudden onset of pale skin and unconsciousness. The heart monitor showed a rapid, uncoordinated activity of the ventricles. The paramedics administered an electric shock by automated defibrillator with the aim of restoring the normal heart rhythm, which is called a(n) _____

2. In the hospital emergency room, Mr. B was given medications by vein to restore blood flow to the damaged tissues of the heart. The lack of blood flow results in damage to the middle layer of the heart wall, tissue known as the _____

3. The recording of the electrical activity of Mr. B's heart indicated that the conduction system was damaged. He was scheduled to have a device inserted to supply impulses needed to stimulate heart contractions. This device is called a(n) _____

4. Mr. P, age 52, had been having episodes of pain in the chest and left shoulder known as angina pectoris, which was not controlled with nitroglycerin. He was scheduled for a procedure in which a catheter with a balloon is used to open up narrow vessels in the heart. This procedure is called _____

5. Baby G's mother brought him into the pediatrician's office. The infant looked small and thin except for a large abdomen. He had not gained the expected amount of weight. His skin was dusky, and the physician heard a loud heart murmur. Further testing indicated an opening between the right and left ventricle. The most common congenital heart defect occurs in this area, which is known as the _____

IX. Short Essays

1. Explain why the heart is described as a double pump.

_____

_____

_____

2. Although the heartbeat originates within the heart itself, it is influenced by factors in the internal environment. Describe some of these factors that can affect the heart.

_____

_____

_____

3. List some modifiable factors that may reduce the risk of heart disease.

_____

_____

_____

15

Blood Vessels and Blood Circulation

Overview

The blood vessels are classified, according to function, as *arteries, veins,* or *capillaries.* Arteries carry blood away from the heart; veins return blood to the heart. Small arteries are called *arterioles,* and small veins are called *venules.* The walls of the arteries are thicker and more elastic than the walls of the veins, and the arteries contain blood under higher pressure. All vessels are lined with a single layer of simple epithelium called *endothelium.* The smallest vessels, the capillaries, are made only of this single layer of cells. It is through the walls of the capillaries that exchanges take place between the blood and the tissues. Materials move by diffusion as influenced by blood pressure, which pushes fluid out of the capillary, and osmotic pressure, which draws fluid back in.

The vessels carry blood through two circuits. The pulmonary vessels transport blood between the heart and the lungs for gas exchange. The systemic vessels distribute blood high in oxygen to all other body tissues and return deoxygenated blood to the heart.

The walls of the vessels, especially the small arteries, contain smooth muscle that is under the control of the involuntary nervous system. The diameters of the vessels can be regulated by the nervous system to alter blood pressure and to direct blood to various parts of the body as needed. These changes, termed *vasodilation* and *vasoconstriction,* are centrally controlled by a *vasomotor center* in the medulla of the brainstem.

Several forces work together to drive blood back to the heart in the venous system. Contraction of skeletal muscles compresses the veins and pushes blood forward, valves in the veins keep blood from flowing backward, and changes in pressure that occur during breathing help to drive blood back to the heart. The

pulse rate and ***blood pressure*** are manifestations of the circulation; they tell the
trained person a great deal about the overall condition of an individual.
  Disorders of the circulatory system include hypertension, degenerative changes
or obstructions that diminish blood flow in the vessels, and hemorrhage.

II. Topics for Review

A. Blood vessels
    1. Types
    2. Circuits
    3. Structure
B. Systemic arteries
    1. Branches of the aorta
    2. Branches of the iliac arteries
    3. Other parts of the arterial system
    4. Anastomoses
C. Systemic veins
    1. Superficial
    2. Deep
    3. Superior and inferior venae cavae
    4. Sinuses
    5. The hepatic portal system
D. Circulation physiology
    1. Capillary exchange
    2. Vasodilation and vasoconstriction
    3. Return of blood to the heart

E. Pulse
F. Blood pressure
　　1. Factors that affect blood pressure
　　2. Measurement
G. Disorders of blood vessels

III. Matching Exercises

Matching only within each group, write the answers in the spaces provided.

Group A

aorta	endothelium	pulmonary circuit
artery	carotid arteries	celiac trunk
systemic circuit	capillary	coronary arteries

1. The tissue that comprises the innermost layer of a blood vessel　　_____

2. The vessels that supply the head and neck on each side　　_____

3. The group of vessels that carries nutrients and oxygen to all tissues of the body except the lungs　　_____

4. A short, unpaired artery that supplies some of the viscera of the upper abdomen　　_____

5. A blood vessel that carries blood away from the heart　　_____

6. The group of vessels that carries blood to and from the lungs for gas exchange　　_____

7. The vessels that branch off the ascending aorta and supply the heart muscle　　_____

8. The largest artery in the body　　_____

9. A small vessel through which exchanges between the blood and the cells take place　　_____

Group B

anastomosis	portal system	vasomotor center
valve	arteriole	blood pressure
venule		

1. A communication between two blood vessels　　_____

2. An area of the medulla that controls dilation and constriction of the blood vessels　　_____

3. A vessel that receives blood from the capillaries　　_____

4. A force that drives materials out of the capillaries　　_____

5. A small artery _____

6. Structure that prevents blood from moving backward
   in the veins _____

7. Term for a circuit that carries venous blood to a second
   capillary bed before it returns to the heart _____

Group C

phrenic artery   lumbar arteries   brachial artery
superior mesenteric artery   right subclavian artery   left common carotid artery
renal arteries   hepatic artery   brachiocephalic trunk
common iliac arteries

1. A short artery that branches off the aortic arch and
   carries blood toward the head and the right arm _____

2. A vessel that supplies the diaphragm _____

3. The vessels that supply blood to the abdominal wall _____

4. The vessel that carries oxygenated blood to the liver _____

5. The large, paired branches of the abdominal aorta that
   supply blood to the kidneys _____

6. The branch of the brachiocephalic artery that supplies
   blood to the right upper extremity _____

7. The largest branch of the abdominal aorta, a vessel that
   supplies most of the small intestine and the first half
   of the large intestine _____

8. The vessels formed by final division of the abdominal aorta _____

9. The vessel that supplies the left side of the head and neck _____

10. The main vessel that supplies the arm, a continuation of
    the axillary artery supplying the arm _____

Group D

circle of Willis   radial artery   basilar artery
mesenteric arches   femoral artery   brachiocephalic trunk
celiac trunk   volar arch

1. The vessel formed by union of the two vertebral arteries _____

2. The anastomosis formed by the radial and ulnar
   arteries in the hand _____

3. The branch of the brachial artery that extends down
   the thumb side of the forearm and wrist _____

4. The short artery that branches into the left gastric artery, the splenic artery, and the hepatic artery _____

5. An anastomosis under the center of the brain formed by two internal carotid arteries and the basilar artery _____

6. The large vessel that branches into the right subclavian artery and the right common carotid artery _____

7. The vessel in the thigh that is a continuation of the external iliac artery _____

8. Anastomoses between branches of the vessels supplying blood to the intestinal tract _____

Group E

azygos vein	median cubital vein	saphenous vein
inferior vena cava	hepatic portal vein	superior vena cava
jugular vein	brachiocephalic vein	venous sinus

1. A large channel that drains deoxygenated blood _____

2. The vein that drains the area supplied by the carotid artery _____

3. The vessel formed by union of the jugular and subclavian veins _____

4. A vessel that drains blood from the chest wall and empties into the superior vena cava _____

5. The vein that receives blood draining from the head, the neck, upper extremities, and the chest _____

6. The vein that receives blood from the unpaired abdominal organs and enters the liver _____

7. The large vein that drains blood from the parts of the body below the diaphragm _____

8. A vein frequently used for removing blood for testing because of its location near the surface at the front of the elbow _____

9. The longest vein _____

Group F

superior sagittal sinus	hepatic veins	left testicular vein
coronary sinus	transverse sinuses	cavernous sinus
common iliac veins	sinusoids	gastric veins
superior mesenteric vein		

1. The channel that receives blood from most of the veins of the heart wall

_____

2. A paired vein that empties into the renal vein instead of emptying directly into the vena cava

_____

3. The channel that drains blood from the ophthalmic vein of the eye

_____

4. The vein that drains most of the small intestine and the first part of the large intestine

_____

5. The veins that drain the stomach and empty into the hepatic portal vein

_____

6. The two veins that unite to form the inferior vena cava

_____

7. A long, blood-filled space in the midline above the brain and in the fissure between the two cerebral hemispheres

_____

8. Enlarged capillary channels where exchanges take place within the liver

_____

9. The paired veins that drain the liver and empty directly into the inferior vena cava

_____

10. The large lateral spaces between the layers of the dura mater that eventually receive nearly all the blood from the brain

_____

Group G

coronary artery	femoral artery	radial artery
saphenous vein	brachial artery	facial artery
dorsalis pedis	cerebral artery	

1. A vessel that may be compressed against the lower jaw to stop hemorrhage around the nose and mouth

_____

2. A vessel that supplies the brain

_____

3. A vessel that supplies the heart muscle

_____

4. The artery in the groin that is compressed to stop hemorrhage of the lower extremity

_____

5. The vessel that is compressed along the groove between the two large arm muscles to stop hemorrhage from the forearm, wrist, and hand

_____

6. The artery on the top of the foot that is sometimes
   used for obtaining the pulse   _____

7. The artery that passes over the bone on the thumb side
   of the wrist and is often used to measure the pulse   _____

8. A large vessel from the thigh that often is used
   for a bypass graft   _____

Group H

aneurysm	arteriosclerosis	atherosclerosis
systolic	hypertension	sphygmomanometer
hypotension	diastolic	pulse

1. Term for the blood pressure reading taken during
   ventricular relaxation   _____

2. A wave of increased pressure that begins at the heart
   when the ventricles contract and travels along the arteries   _____

3. The condition in which calcium salts and fibrous
   connective tissues infiltrate the artery walls and
   cause hardening of the arteries   _____

4. An abnormal increase in blood pressure   _____

5. An instrument that is used to measure blood pressure   _____

6. Term for blood pressure measured during heart
   muscle contraction   _____

7. An abnormal decrease in blood pressure, as may
   occur in shock   _____

8. A change in the arterial walls in which yellow, fatlike
   material replaces muscle and elastic connective tissue   _____

9. A bulging sac in the wall of an artery that results
   from weakness of the vessel wall   _____

IV. Multiple Choice

Select the best answer and write the letter of your choice in the blank.

1. Which of the following is *not* a subdivision of the aorta?   1. _____

   a. thoracic aorta
   b. descending aorta
   c. aortic arch
   d. pulmonary aorta
   e. abdominal aorta

2. Which of the following arteries is unpaired?

    a. common carotid
    b. brachiocephalic
    c. external iliac
    d. brachial
    e. renal

2. _____

3. Which of the following arteries carries blood low in oxygen?

    a. hepatic artery
    b. hepatic portal artery
    c. brachiocephalic artery
    d. superior vena cava
    e. pulmonary artery

3. _____

4. The intercostal arteries are located

    a. in the inguinal region
    b. below the kidneys
    c. between the ribs
    d. in the groin
    e. between the arm and forearm

4. _____

5. Tissue fluid is also called

    a. venous fluid
    b. interstitial fluid
    c. plasma
    d. sinus fluid
    e. lymph

5. _____

6. The precapillary sphincter is a

    a. ring of smooth muscle that regulates blood flow
    b. dilated vein in the liver
    c. small artery in the brain
    d. damaged valve in a vessel
    e. valve at the entrance to the iliac artery

6. _____

7. The term *viscosity* means

    a. solubility
    b. rate
    c. dilation
    d. thickness
    e. volume

7. _____

8. The middle layer of the arterial wall is composed of elastic connective tissue and

    a. cartilage
    b. endothelium
    c. smooth muscle
    d. adipose tissue
    e. skeletal muscle

8. _____

9. As blood flows through the tissues, a force that draws fluid
   back into the capillaries is

   a. blood pressure
   b. osmotic pressure
   c. hypertension
   d. vasoconstriction
   e. systolic pressure

9. _____

10. A piece of a clot that breaks loose and travels in the vessels is a(n)

    a. aneurysm
    b. septic shock
    c. inflammation of a vein
    d. plaque
    e. embolus

10. _____

11. Necrosis is

    a. loss of oxygen
    b. death of tissue
    c. accumulation of wastes
    d. narrowing of a vessel
    e. hardening of the arteries

11. _____

12. A swollen and ineffective vein is described as

    a. varicose
    b. sclerotic
    c. anastomosed
    d. constricted
    e. anaphylactic

12. _____

V. Labeling

For each of the following illustrations, write the name or names of each labeled part on the numbered lines.

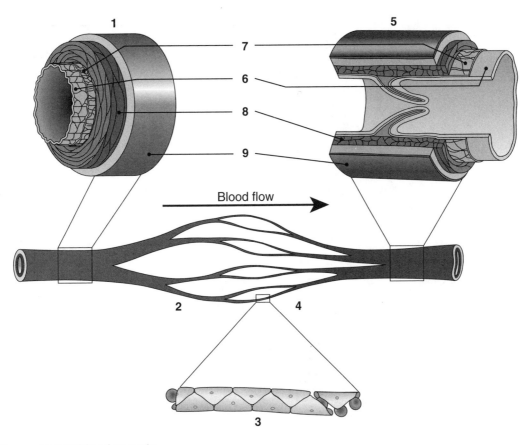

Blood flow

Sections of small blood vessels

1. _____   6. _____

2. _____   7. _____

3. _____   8. _____

4. _____   9. _____

5. _____

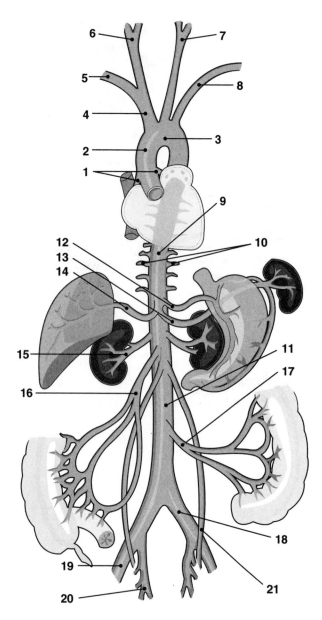

Aorta and its branches

1. _____
2. _____
3. _____
4. _____
5. _____
6. _____
7. _____
8. _____
9. _____
10. _____
11. _____
12. _____
13. _____
14. _____
15. _____
16. _____
17. _____
18. _____
19. _____
20. _____
21. _____

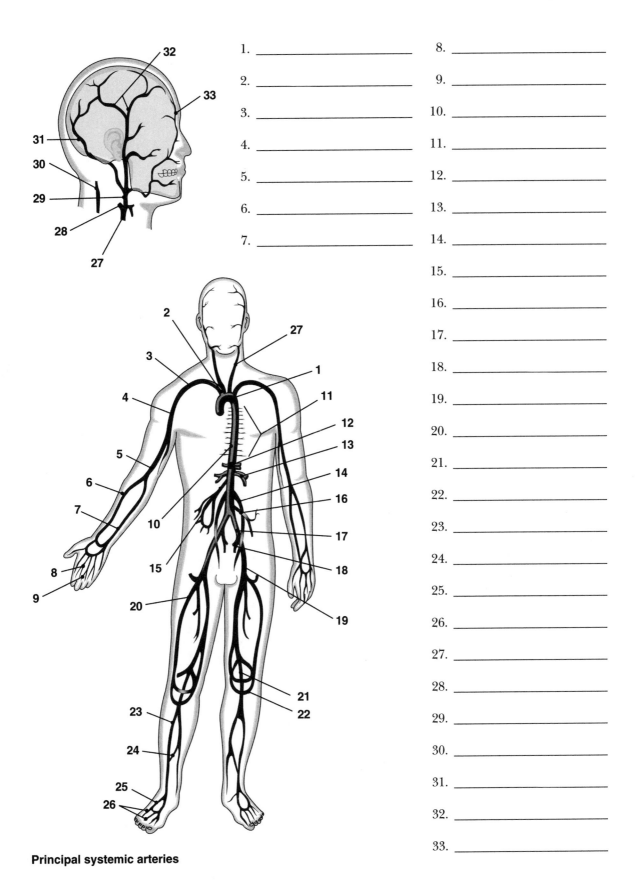

1. _____

2. _____

3. _____

4. _____

5. _____

6. _____

7. _____

8. _____

9. _____

10. _____

11. _____

12. _____

13. _____

14. _____

15. _____

16. _____

17. _____

18. _____

19. _____

20. _____

21. _____

22. _____

23. _____

24. _____

25. _____

26. _____

27. _____

28. _____

29. _____

30. _____

31. _____

32. _____

33. _____

Principal systemic arteries

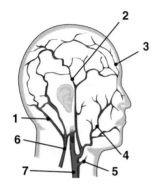

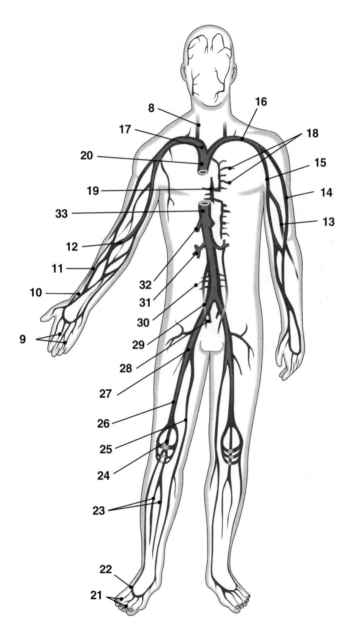

Principal systemic veins

1. _____

2. _____

3. _____

4. _____

5. _____

6. _____

7. _____

8. _____

9. _____

10. _____

11. _____

12. _____

13. _____

14. _____

15. _____

16. _____

17. _____

18. _____

19. _____

20. _____

21. _____

22. _____

23. _____

24. _____

25. _____

26. _____

27. _____

28. _____

29. _____

30. _____

31. _____

32. _____

33. _____

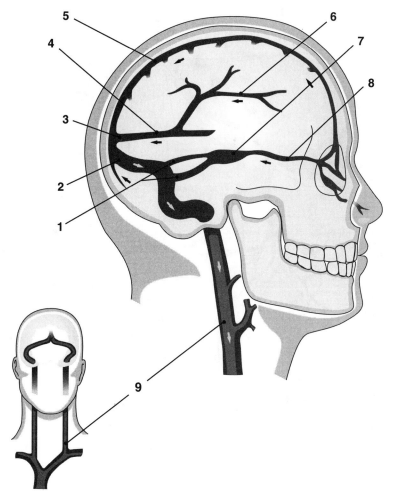

Cranial venous sinuses

1. _____

2. _____

3. _____

4. _____

5. _____

6. _____

7. _____

8. _____

9. _____

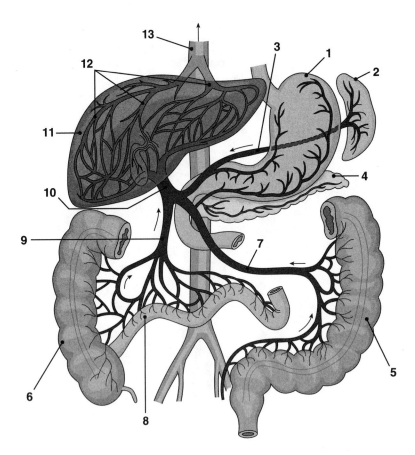

Hepatic portal circulation

1. _____   8. _____

2. _____   9. _____

3. _____   10. _____

4. _____   11. _____

5. _____   12. _____

6. _____   13. _____

7. _____

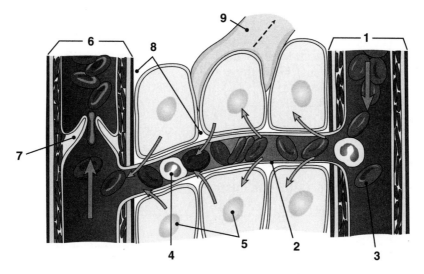

Connection between small blood vessels

1. _____   6. _____

2. _____   7. _____

3. _____   8. _____

4. _____   9. _____

5. _____

VI. True–False

For each question, write T for true or F for false in the blank to the left of each number. If a statement is false, correct it by replacing the underlined term and write the correct statement in the blanks below the question.

_____ 1. A small vein is called a <u>capillary</u>.

_____

_____

_____ 2. The thoracic aorta supplies structures in the <u>chest</u>.

_____

_____

_____ 3. <u>Veins</u> carry blood toward the heart.

_____

_____

_____ 4. The widening of a blood vessel is termed <u>vasoconstriction</u>.

_____

_____

_____ 5. The circle of Willis is an anastomosis of vessels supplying blood to the <u>heart.</u>

_____

_____

_____ 6. The iliac veins empty into the <u>superior vena cava</u>.

_____

_____

_____ 7. Another name for high blood pressure is <u>hypotension</u>.

_____

_____

_____ 8. <u>Diastolic</u> pressure is measured when the heart relaxes.

_____

_____

_____ 9. The liver is supplied with oxygenated blood through the <u>hepatic portal vein.</u>

_____

_____

_____ 10. Phlebitis is inflammation of a <u>vein.</u>

_____

_____

VII. Completion Exercise

Write the word or phrase that correctly completes each sentence.

1. The vessel that receives blood from the left ventricle is the _____

2. The special type of epithelium that lines the blood vessels and makes up the capillaries is _____

3. Deoxygenated blood is carried from the right ventricle by the _____

4. The smallest subdivisions of arteries have thin walls in which there is little connective tissue and relatively more muscle. These vessels are _____

5. Supplying nutrients to all body tissues except the lungs and carrying off waste products from these tissues are functions of the vascular circuit described as the _____

6. The wave of increased pressure that can be felt in the arteries as the heart contracts is the _____

7. A life-threatening condition in which there is inadequate blood flow to the tissues due to inadequate output by the heart is _____

8. Hemorrhoids are varicose veins located in the _____

9. People whose work requires them to stand much of the time frequently suffer from varicosities of the long leg veins named the _____

10. The circle of Willis is formed by a union of the internal carotid arteries and the basilar artery. Such a union of vessels is called a(n) _____

11. One example of a portal system is the system that carries blood from the abdominal organs to the _____

VIII. Practical Applications

Study each discussion. Then write the appropriate word or phrase in the space provided.

Group A

1. Mr. S, age 53, complained of shortness of breath, weakness, and pain in the left chest. Examination indicated that the left semilunar valve was not functioning properly. This valve guards the entrance into the largest artery, which is the

   _____

2. Mrs. K, age 69, was brought to the hospital emergency department due to episodes of fainting and loss of consciousness. She had a history of diabetes and hypertension and was unable to remember events surrounding this latest episode of fainting. An examination of the blood vessels in the eye and an ultrasound of the carotid arteries showed damage and narrowing of blood vessels. The physician diagnosed the most common type of arterial damage, which is known as

   _____

3. In cases such as Mrs. K's, the gradual narrowing of the arteries in the brain leads to a reduction in the volume of blood flowing to the tissues. This lack of blood to the tissues is called

   _____

4. When the blood supply to an organ is inadequate, the cells of that organ gradually die. Cell death is called

   _____

Group B

1. Ms. J, age 78, complained of pain and swelling in the area of her saphenous vein. The term for venous inflammation is

   _____

2. Further study of Ms. J's illness indicated that in association with the inflammation a blood clot had formed in one vein. This serious condition is called

   _____

3. Ms. J was put on bedrest with her legs elevated and was started on anticoagulant medications. These measures were taken to reduce the serious risk that the blood clot would break loose and travel to the lungs. This potentially fatal complication is called

   _____

4. John J, injured in an automobile accident, was brought to the emergency room bleeding profusely from several lacerations. This type of bleeding is called

   _____

5. Mr. B, age 67, had been diabetic for the past several years. He had neglected his diet and was careless about following his physician's orders. Now, the physician found it necessary to order amputation of his right foot because necrosis and infection of the involved tissue had resulted in a condition called

   _____

6. Mr. W was seen in the hospital emergency room. He complained of severe, crushing chest pain. Further observation yielded these objective signs: pulse of 120, weak; blood pressure 76/40; skin cold, clammy, and gray; rapid, shallow respiration. His symptoms were due to failure of the heart pump, a form of shock known as

   _____

7. Mrs. H, age 72, a clinic patient with a history of varicose veins, was being examined because of the presence of an open sore on her lower leg. The skin surrounding the sore was scaling, inflamed, and cracked, all symptoms of a type of ulcer called

   _____

IX. Short Essays

1. Explain the purpose of vascular anastomoses.

   _____

   _____

   _____

2. What is the function of the hepatic portal system, and what vessels contribute to this system?

   _____

   _____

   _____

3. Explain how the structure of the capillaries allows them to function in exchanges between the blood and the tissues.

   _____

   _____

   _____

4. Describe the forces that influence blood pressure.

   _____

   _____

   _____

16 The Lymphatic System and Lymphoid Tissue

I. Overview

Lymph is the watery fluid that flows within the lymphatic system. It originates from the blood plasma and from the tissue fluid that is found in the minute spaces around and between the body cells. The fluid moves from the *lymphatic capillaries* through the *lymphatic vessels* and then to the *right lymphatic duct* and the *thoracic duct.* These large terminal ducts drain into the subclavian veins, adding the lymph to blood that is returning to the heart. Lymphatic capillaries resemble blood capillaries, but they begin blindly and larger gaps between the cells make them more permeable than blood capillaries. The larger lymphatic vessels are thin-walled and delicate; like some veins, they have valves that prevent backflow of lymph.

The *lymph nodes,* which are the system's filters, are composed of lymphoid *tissue.* These nodes remove impurities and process *lymphocytes,* cells active in immunity. Chief among them are the cervical nodes in the neck, the axillary nodes in the armpit, the tracheobronchial nodes near the trachea and bronchial tubes, the mesenteric nodes between the peritoneal layers, and the inguinal nodes in the groin.

In addition to the nodes, there are several organs of lymphoid tissue with somewhat different functions. The *tonsils* filter tissue fluid; the *thymus* is essential for development of the immune system during early life. The *spleen* has numerous functions, including destruction of worn out red blood cells, serving as a reservoir for blood, and producing red blood cells before birth.

Another part of the body's protective system is the *reticuloendothelial system,* which consists of cells involved in the destruction of bacteria, cancer cells, and other possibly harmful substances.

Disorders of the lymphatic system include inflammation and enlargement of lymphoid tissue, neoplastic diseases, and elephantiasis, caused by a worm.

II. Topics for Review

A. Lymph
B. Lymphatic vessels
C. Lymphatic tissue
   1. Lymph nodes
   2. Tonsils
   3. Thymus
   4. Spleen
D. The reticuloendothelial system
E. Disorders of the lymphatic system

III. Matching Exercises

Matching only within each group, write the answers in the spaces provided.

Group A

inguinal nodes	thymus	axillary nodes
endothelium	right lymphatic duct	chyle
cervical nodes		

1. The vessel that drains lymph from the right side of the body
   above the diaphragm   _____

2. The milky-appearing fluid that is a combination of fat globules and lymph

_____

3. The special single layer of cells that makes up the walls of lymphatic capillaries and blood capillaries

_____

4. The lymph nodes located in the neck that drain certain parts of the head and neck

_____

5. The lymph nodes located in the armpits

_____

6. A lymphoid structure that is essential in the development of immunity very early in life

_____

7. The nodes that filter lymph from the lower extremities and the external genitalia

_____

Group B

palatine tonsils   valves   spleen
lymphangitis   lingual tonsils   pharyngeal tonsil
lacteals   lymphadenitis

1. An inflammatory disorder of lymph nodes

_____

2. Specialized lymphatic capillaries of the intestine that absorb digested fats

_____

3. The oval lymphoid bodies located at each side of the soft palate

_____

4. The organ that filters blood and is located in the upper left quadrant (left hypochondriac region) of the abdomen

_____

5. Inflammation of lymphatic vessels

_____

6. Masses of lymphoid tissue at the back of the tongue

_____

7. The mass of lymphoid tissue located in the pharynx behind the nose and commonly called adenoids

_____

8. Structures that prevent backflow of fluid in lymphatic vessels

_____

Group C

monocytes   antibodies   subclavian vein
femoral   thymus   phagocytosis
thoracic duct   mesenteric

1. The blood vessel on the right side of the body that receives lymph from the right lymphatic duct

_____

2. The large lymphatic vessel that drains lymph from below the diaphragm and from the left side above the diaphragm

_____

3. The white blood cells that give rise to macrophages, cells active in the reticuloendothelial system

_____

4. Term for lymphatic vessels in the thigh

_____

5. The process by which cells engulf foreign substances, such as bacteria

_____

6. The organ in which T cells mature

_____

7. Substances produced by lymphocytes that aid in combating infection

_____

8. Term for lymph nodes located between the layers of the peritoneum

_____

Group D

cisterna chyli	buboes	proteins
lymph	filariae	plasma
superficial	veins	

1. The small parasitic worms that cause elephantiasis

_____

2. The temporary storage area formed by an enlargement of the first part of the thoracic duct

_____

3. The vessels that often accompany the deep vessels of the lymphatic system

_____

4. Abnormally large inguinal nodes, as may be found in certain infections

_____

5. The liquid part of the blood that gives rise to intercellular fluid

_____

6. The fluid formed when tissue fluid passes from the intercellular spaces into the lymphatic vessels

_____

7. Term for lymphatic vessels located under the skin

_____

8. Substances absorbed from tissue fluid into the lymph to be returned to the blood

_____

Group E

Kupffer's cells	hilum	thoracic duct
spleen	chyle	macrophages

1. A lymphoid organ that produces red blood cells during embryonic and fetal life

_____

2. The name for monocytes that enter the body tissues and
   act to destroy foreign matter

   _____

3. The phagocytes of the liver

   _____

4. The larger of the terminal vessels of the lymphatic system

   _____

5. The area of exit for the vessels carrying lymph out of a node

   _____

6. The fluid that drains into the lacteals of the small intestine

   _____

IV. Multiple Choice

Select the best answer and write the letter of your choice in the blank.

1. The blockage of lymphatic vessels by filariae may cause
   tremendous enlargement of the lower extremities, a disorder called

   1. _____

   a. septicemia
   b. lymphosarcoma
   c. elephantiasis
   d. lymphadenopathy
   e. non-Hodgkin's lymphoma

2. Which of the following is *not* a type of cell associated with
   the reticuloendothelial system?

   2. _____

   a. monocytes
   b. red blood cells
   c. macrophages
   d. Kupffer's cells
   e. dust cells

3. Thymosin is

   3. _____

   a. the hormone produced by the thymus gland
   b. enlargement of the lymph nodes
   c. the fluid in the lymphatic vessels
   d. the fluid that drains from the intestine into the lymphatic system
   e. the hormone produced by the thyroid gland

4. Which of the following is *not* a function of the spleen?

   4. _____

   a. destruction of old red blood cells
   b. filtration of blood
   c. storage of blood
   d. drainage of chyle
   e. phagocytosis

5. Splenomegaly is

   5. _____

   a. rupture of the spleen
   b. removal of the spleen
   c. communication between the spleen and liver
   d. infection of the spleen
   e. enlargement of the spleen

6. An organ that shrinks in size after puberty is the

    a. lacteal
    b. cisterna chyli
    c. lymph node
    d. liver
    e. thymus

6. _____

7. Enlargement of the lymph nodes, as seen in Hodgkin's disease, AIDS, and infectious mononucleosis, is termed

    a. tonsillitis
    b. lymphadenopathy
    c. lymphangitis
    d. adenoidectomy
    e. splenectomy

7. _____

V. Labeling

For each of the following illustrations, write the name or names of each labeled part on the numbered lines.

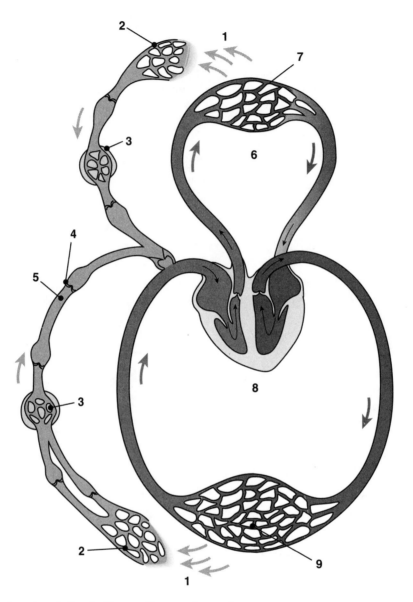

Lymphatic system in relation to the cardiovascular system

1. _____

2. _____

3. _____

4. _____

5. _____

6. _____

7. _____

8. _____

9. _____

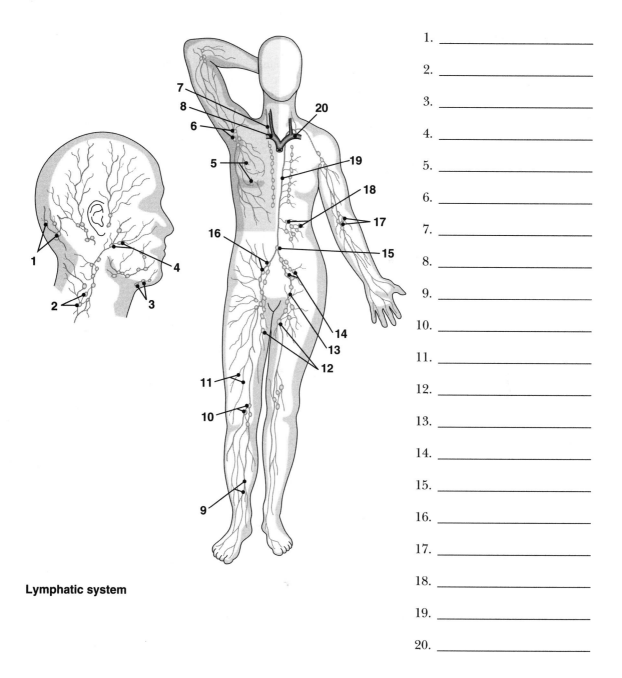

Lymphatic system

1. _____

2. _____

3. _____

4. _____

5. _____

6. _____

7. _____

8. _____

9. _____

10. _____

11. _____

12. _____

13. _____

14. _____

15. _____

16. _____

17. _____

18. _____

19. _____

20. _____

VI. True–False

For each question, write T for true or F for false in the blank to the left of each number. If a statement is false, correct it by replacing the underlined term and write the correct statement in the blanks below the question.

_____ 1. The <u>superficial</u> lymphatic vessels are near the surface of the body.

_____

_____

_____ 2. The <u>inguinal</u> lymph nodes are in the groin.

_____

_____

_____ 3. The <u>thoracic duct</u> drains the lower part of the body and the upper left portion of the body.

_____

_____

_____ 4. Lacteals are located in the <u>stomach</u>.

_____

_____

_____ 5. The large lymphatic vessels empty into the <u>subclavian arteries</u>.

_____

_____

_____ 6. The lymph nodes located in the neck are the <u>axillary</u> nodes.

_____

_____

_____ 7. <u>Adenoids</u> is a common name for the <u>pharyngeal tonsil</u>.

_____

_____

VII. Completion Exercise

Write the word or phrase that correctly completes each sentence.

1. The fluid that moves from tissue spaces into special collection vessels for return to the blood is called _____

2. The word root *angi-*, meaning "vessel" is found in the term for inflammation of lymphatic vessels. This term is _____

3. Lymphatic vessels from the left side of the head, neck, and thorax empty into the largest of the lymphatic vessels, the _____

4. Lymph from the right side of the body above the diaphragm joins the bloodstream when the right lymphatic duct empties into the _____

5. The milky-appearing lymph that drains from the small intestine is called _____

6. Among those living in highly polluted areas, the lymph nodes surrounding the breathing passageways may become black with carbon particles. The nodes involved are the _____

7. A disease prevalent in the Middle Ages was responsible for the death of hundreds of thousands of people. This disease was characterized by the presence of buboes, inflammatory swellings of the inguinal nodes, so it was called _____

8. Some specialized blood cells can engulf harmful bacteria and other foreign cells by a process called _____

9. A tumor that occurs in lymphoid tissue, whether benign or malignant, has the general name of _____

VIII. Practical Applications

Study each discussion. Then write the appropriate word or phrase in the space provided.

1. Mrs. B, age 52, a patient with a breast mass biopsy positive for malignancy was scheduled for surgery. The surgeon was planning to remove the breast and most of the lymph nodes in the armpit to prevent the spread of the disease. The lymph nodes located in the armpit are called the _____

2. Mr. G, age 31, complained of swellings in his neck, his armpits, his groin, and other areas. A diagnosis of Hodgkin's disease was made. The nodes of the neck are designated the _____

3. Mr. K, age 27, was seen by his physician with a history of fevers, night sweats, and enlarged lymph nodes. He was sent to the laboratory for a number of blood tests to differentiate between several disorders that cause enlargement of the lymph nodes. Pending the results of the laboratory tests, the physician called the painless enlargement of the lymph nodes _____

4. Mrs. M had undergone a series of diagnostic tests to determine the cause of her enlarged spleen. This condition of the spleen is called _____

5. After her tests were completed, Mrs. M was found to have the diagnosis of hemolytic anemia. This disease can be controlled by removal of the spleen, an operation called a(n) _____

6. Mr. L, age 58, was in the outpatient surgery department to have a biopsy as part of a series of specialized tests to determine the cause of his pelvic mass. He also had enlarged cervical nodes and other indications that his disease was widespread. The tentative diagnosis was a malignancy of the lymphatic system called _____

7. Mr. J was 21 years old. His complaint concerned swelling in the groin region. A blood test showed that the young man had contracted syphilis. Infection of the external genitalia is often followed by the appearance of buboes, which are enlarged _____

IX. Short Essays

1. Compare lymphatic capillaries and blood capillaries.

_____

_____

_____

2. Describe the mechanisms that move lymph forward in the lymphatic vessels.

_____

_____

_____

3. What is the function of the reticuloendothelial system? Give several examples of cells that function in this system.

_____

_____

_____

17

Body Defense, Immunity, and Vaccines

I. Overview

Although the body is constantly being exposed to pathogenic organisms, infection develops relatively rarely. This is because the body has many "lines of defense" against pathogenic invasion. The intact *skin* and *mucous membranes* serve as mechanical barriers, as do certain *reflexes* such as sneezing and coughing. Body secretions wash away impurities and may kill bacteria as well. By the process of *inflammation,* the body tries to get rid of an irritant or to minimize its harmful effects. *Phagocytes* and *natural killer (NK) cells* act nonspecifically to destroy invaders. *Interferon* can limit viral infections. *Fever* boosts the immune system and inhibits the growth of some organisms.

The ultimate defense against disease is *immunity,* the means by which the body resists or overcomes the effects of a particular disease or other harmful agent. There are two basic types of immunity: inborn and acquired. *Inborn immunity* is inherited; it may exist on the basis of *species, population,* or *individual* characteristics. *Acquired immunity* is gained during a person's lifetime. It involves reactions between foreign substances or *antigens* and the white blood cells known as *lymphocytes.* The *T cells* (T lymphocytes) respond to the antigen directly and produce *cell-mediated immunity.* There are different types of T cells involved in immune reactions, some acting to control the response. *Macrophages* participate by presenting the foreign antigen to the T cell. *B cells* (B lymphocytes), when stimulated by an antigen, multiply into *plasma cells.* These cells produce specific *antibodies,* which react with the antigen. Circulating antibodies make up the form of immunity termed *humoral immunity.*

Acquired immunity may be *natural* (acquired by transfer of maternal antibodies or by contact with the disease) or *artificial* (provided by a vaccine or an immune serum). Immunity that involves production of antibodies by the individual is termed *active immunity;* immunity acquired as a result of the transfer of antibodies to an individual from some outside source is described as *passive immunity*.

The responses associated with *allergy* (hypersensitivity) are similar to those of immunity, but the reactions are greatly exaggerated. The *rejection syndrome* that often takes place after tissue transplantation is also a natural immune response to foreign tissue. This must be limited by careful cross matching and administration of drugs to suppress the immune system. Research on the immune system has expanded greatly in recent decades. Areas of interest include the study of HIV, the virus that causes acquired immunodeficiency syndrome (AIDS); study of the role of the immune system in cancer; and study of autoimmune diseases.

II. Topics for Review

A. Nonspecific defenses against disease
   1. Chemical and mechanical barriers
   2. Phagocytosis
   3. Natural killer (NK) cells
   4. Inflammation
   5. Fever
   6. Interferon
B. Specific defenses: immunity
   1. Inborn
   2. Acquired
      a. Natural or artificial
      b. Active or passive

C. The immune response
   1. Lymphocytes (T cells and B cells)
   2. Antigens
   3. Antibodies
D. Vaccines and immunization
E. Disorders involving the immune system
   1. Allergy
   2. Autoimmunity
   3. Immune deficiency
   4. Transplantation and the rejection syndrome

III. Matching Exercises

Matching only within each group, write the answers in the spaces provided.

Group A

interferon	virulence	portal of entry
immunity	NK cell	thymus
toxin	mucous membranes	

1. The body's specific defense against certain agents of disease _____

2. A lymphocyte that nonspecifically destroys abnormal cells _____

3. The organ to which T cells migrate when they leave the bone marrow _____

4. The means by which a pathogenic organism invades the body _____

5. A poison produced by a pathogen _____

6. The tissues invaded by the viruses that cause the common cold and influenza _____

7. The power of an organism to overcome body defenses and cause disease _____

8. A substance that prevents multiplication of viruses _____

Group B

B cells	attenuation	active immunity
antigen	passive immunity	species immunity
inflammation	macrophages	

1. Any foreign substance introduced into the body that provokes an immune response _____

2. The lymphocytes that multiply in response to infection, giving rise to cells that produce antibodies _____

3. The type of protection that prevents humans from contracting certain animal diseases _____

4. A nonspecific response by which the body tries to get rid of (or minimize the effects of) an irritant

   _____

5. The type of long-term immunity produced by infection or exposure to a microbial toxin

   _____

6. The process of reducing the virulence of a pathogen to prepare a vaccine

   _____

7. The type of immunity that results from transfer of antibodies from mother to fetus through the placenta

   _____

8. Cells derived from monocytes that work with T cells

   _____

Group C

complement	histamine	immunization
memory cell	plasma cell	gamma globulin
allergy	toxoid	

1. A toxin treated with heat or chemicals to reduce its harmfulness so that it may be used as a vaccine

   _____

2. A group of blood proteins that may be needed to help an antibody destroy a foreign antigen

   _____

3. An antibody-producing cell derived from a B cell

   _____

4. Use of a vaccine to protect against infection

   _____

5. The type of lymphocyte that is stimulated by a booster shot

   _____

6. A tendency to react unfavorably to substances that are normally harmless to most people

   _____

7. The fraction of the blood plasma that contains antibodies

   _____

8. A substance released from damaged tissue

   _____

Group D

urticaria	allergen	antivenin
hypersensitivity	autoimmunity	transplantation
rubella	antitoxin	antibody

1. Another term for allergy

   _____

2. The manufacture of antibodies to one's own tissues

   _____

3. The type of antiserum that is injected to combat the effects of poisonous snake bites

   _____

4. The grafting of tissue from one person to another

   _____

5. The type of immune serum used to provide passive immunity to diphtheria

_____

6. The substance in an immune serum that is active against a disease organism

_____

7. A disorder that may cause serious effects on the developing fetus

_____

8. A protein that stimulates an allergic response, as is found in pollen and house dust

_____

9. Another name for hives

_____

IV. Multiple Choice

Select the best answer and write the letter of your choice in the blank.

1. The mixture of leukocytes and fluid from the blood plasma that is produced as the body tries to defend itself against pathogens is known as the inflammatory

1. _____

   a. serum
   b. exudate
   c. interferon
   d. complement
   e. antibody

2. Which of the following is a specific defense against infection?

2. _____

   a. skin
   b. tears
   c. mucus
   d. antibodies
   e. cilia

3. The condition of the individual that leads to disease is his or her

3. _____

   a. exposure
   b. dose
   c. predisposition
   d. virulence
   e. resistance

4. MHC antigens are

4. _____

   a. bacterial proteins
   b. antibodies
   c. foreign proteins
   d. a type of mucus
   e. one's own proteins

5. Cells that combine with foreign antigens and present them to the T cells are the

    a. allergens
    b. B cells
    c. macrophages
    d. lymphocytes
    e. viruses

5. _____

6. Interleukins are

    a. a group of nonspecific proteins needed for agglutination
    b. substances in the blood that react with antigens
    c. the antibody fraction of the blood
    d. substances released from macrophages that stimulate T cells
    e. a type of immune serum

6. _____

7. Which of the following does *not* describe an activity of T cells?

    a. helping other immune cells to act
    b. suppression of the immune response
    c. manufacture of antibodies
    d. direct destruction of foreign cells
    e. remembering an antigen for future response

7. _____

8. Booster shots are given to

    a. maintain antibody titers
    b. transfer antibodies passively
    c. cross match for transplantation
    d. avoid serum sickness
    e. reduce the immune response

8. _____

V. True–False

For each question, write T for true or F for false in the blank to the left of each number. If a statement is false, correct it by replacing the underlined term and write the correct statement in the blanks below the question.

_____ 1. Most antigens are proteins.

_____

_____

_____ 2. The skin, mucous membranes, and secretions that destroy bacteria are examples of nonspecific defenses.

_____

_____

_____ 3. The poliomyelitis virus attacks <u>nervous tissue.</u>

_____

_____

_____ 4. Immunity produced by transfer of antibodies from one person to another is described as <u>active</u> immunity.

_____

_____

_____ 5. Antigen-presenting cells are <u>macrophages.</u>

_____

_____

_____ 6. T cells produce <u>cell-mediated immunity.</u>

_____

_____

_____ 7. The plasma cells that produce antibodies come from <u>T cells.</u>

_____

_____

_____ 8. Immunoglobulin is another name for <u>antibody.</u>

_____

_____

VI. Completion Exercise

Write the word or phrase that correctly completes each sentence.

1. The power of an organism to overcome the defenses of a host is termed its   _____

2. The action of leukocytes in which they engulf and digest invading pathogens is known as   _____

3. Circulating antibodies are responsible for the type of immunity termed   _____

4. Immunity is a selective process through which a person may be immune to one disease but not to another. This selective characteristic is called

_____

5. There are two main categories of immunity. One is inborn immunity, whereas the other is

_____

6. Heat, redness, swelling, and pain are considered the classic symptoms of

_____

7. Antibodies transmitted from a mother's blood to a fetus provide a type of short-term borrowed immunity called

_____

8. The administration of vaccine, on the other hand, stimulates the body to produce a longer lasting type of immunity called

_____

9. The irritating effects of the allergic response are believed to be an antigen–antibody reaction, which results in the liberation of a substance that dilates the blood vessels and is called

_____

10. The use of methods to stimulate the immune system in the hope of combating cancer is a form of treatment called

_____

11. Transplantation of an organ or tissue may fail because of the recipient's natural tendency to destroy foreign substances, leading to a(n)

_____

VII. Practical Applications

Study each discussion. Then write the appropriate word or phrase in the space provided.

1. Mr. O brought his 38-year-old wife to the local emergency clinic to get treatment for a bee sting. The physician immediately administered an injection of epinephrine to counteract her low blood pressure and difficulty in breathing. Her condition improved rapidly. The physician gave her prescriptions and advice on how to prevent or treat another episode of this disorder, which he termed

_____

2. Mrs. R brought her 2-month-old infant to the office for the first of a series of injections to inoculate him against several serious diseases. The vaccine used for this purpose contains the weakened toxins of the organisms causing these diseases. A vaccine made from an altered toxin is known as a(n)

_____

3. Ms. Y was allergic to pollens. In the hope that her tissues would become desensitized, the physician was giving her repeated injections of the antigen that caused the reaction. The term for an antigen that induces allergy is

_____

4. Mr. N, age 42, had received a kidney transplant. He had appeared well for several months after the operation, when evidence of the rejection syndrome appeared. These reactions are due primarily to the activity of certain white blood cells that defend the body against foreign organisms. They are responsible for cell-mediated immunity and are called _____

5. Mr. S, a construction worker, was careless about cleansing his skin and neglected the abrasions on his fingers. An infection of his right thumb and index finger resulted in painful swelling and prevented him from working. He was treated with hot wet compresses, and in time his natural resistance overcame the infection. To a large extent, this resistance was due to the production of antibodies by the white cells known as _____

6. Mr. K consulted his physician for persistent diarrhea, fever, and enlarged lymph nodes. Blood tests showed that he was infected with a virus that weakened his immune system by destroying certain T cells. The disease caused by this virus is abbreviated to the letters _____

7. Mrs. N was diagnosed as having systemic lupus erythematosus after she consulted her physician for fatigue, skin rashes, and joint pain. Her physician explained that her disease was caused by a reaction of her immune system to her own body proteins, a condition termed _____

VIII. Short Essays

1. The immune system protects against disease. Are there any instances in which this system is harmful to the individual?

   _____

   _____

   _____

2. Describe the factors that influence the occurrence of infection.

   _____

   _____

   _____

3. Explain the role of macrophages in immunity.

   _____

   _____

   _____

Unit VI

ENERGY SUPPLY AND USE

18

Respiration

I. Overview

Oxygen is taken into the body and carbon dioxide is released by means of the organs and passageways that make up the *respiratory system.* This system contains the *nasal cavities,* the *pharynx,* the *larynx,* the *trachea,* the *bronchi,* and the *lungs.*

Oxygen is obtained from the atmosphere and delivered to the cells by the process of *respiration.* The three phases of respiration are: *pulmonary ventilation,* normally accomplished by breathing; *diffusion* of gases between the alveoli of the lungs and the bloodstream; and *transport* of gases in the blood. Oxygen is delivered to the cells, and carbon dioxide is transported to the lungs for elimination.

Oxygen is transported to the tissues almost entirely by the *hemoglobin* in red blood cells. Some carbon dioxide is transported in the red blood cells as well, but most is carried in the blood plasma as the *bicarbonate ion.* Carbon dioxide is important in regulating the pH of the blood and in regulating the breathing rate.

Breathing is primarily controlled by the *respiratory control centers* in the medulla and the pons of the brain stem. These centers are influenced by *chemoreceptors* located outside the medulla that respond to changes in the acidity of the cerebrospinal fluid. There are also *chemoreceptors* in the large vessels of the chest and neck that regulate respiration in response to changes in the composition of the blood.

Disorders of the respiratory tract include infection, allergy, chronic obstructive pulmonary disease (COPD), and cancer.

II. Topics for Review

A. Phases of respiration
B. The respiratory system

C. The process of respiration
   1. Pulmonary ventilation
   2. Gas exchange
   3. Gas transport
   4. Regulation of respiration
   5. Breathing patterns
D. Disorders of the respiratory system

III. Matching Exercises

Matching only within each group, write the answers in the spaces provided.

Group A

diffusion	inhalation	carbon dioxide
exhalation	surfactant	transport
residual volume	respiration	tidal volume

1. The gaseous waste product of cell metabolism   _____

2. The substance in the fluid lining the alveoli that
   prevents their collapse   _____

3. The physical process by which a substance moves from an
   area where it is in higher concentration to an area where
   it is in lower concentration   _____

4. The total process by which oxygen is obtained from the environment and delivered to the cells

   _____

5. The amount of air moved into or out of the lungs in relaxed breathing

   _____

6. The second phase of pulmonary ventilation in which air is expelled from the alveoli

   _____

7. The phase of respiration in which oxygen is carried to the cells by circulating blood

   _____

8. The first phase of pulmonary ventilation in which air is drawn into the lungs

   _____

9. The volume of air that remains in the lungs after maximum exhalation

   _____

Group B

thyroid cartilage   larynx   trachea
pharynx   conchae   nostrils
diaphragm   nasal septum   sinus

1. The scientific name for the windpipe

   _____

2. The scientific name for the cartilaginous structure commonly referred to as the voice box

   _____

3. A small cavity in a bone of the skull lined with mucous membrane

   _____

4. The structure that forms the "Adam's apple"

   _____

5. The muscle that separates the thoracic cavity from the abdominal cavity

   _____

6. The partition separating the two cavities of the nose

   _____

7. The openings of the nose

   _____

8. The three projections arising from the lateral walls of each nasal cavity

   _____

9. The area below the nasal cavities that is common to both the digestive and respiratory systems

   _____

Group C

nasopharynx   epiglottis   cilia
bronchi   esophagus   hilum
vocal cords   oropharynx

1. The leaf-shaped structure that helps to prevent the entrance of food into the trachea

   _____

2. The upper portion of the pharynx

          _____

3. The notch or depression where the bronchus, blood vessels, and nerves enter the lung

          _____

4. The hairlike structures that filter impurities within the conducting tubes of the respiratory tract

          _____

5. The two main air passageways to the lungs, formed by division of the trachea

          _____

6. The structures that vibrate in the air flow from the lungs to aid in production of speech

          _____

7. The tube leading from the pharynx that carries food into the stomach

          _____

8. The portion of the pharynx located behind the mouth

          _____

Group D

hemoglobin   pleura   alveoli
glottis   diaphragm   carbonic anhydrase
bronchiole   mediastinum   carbon dioxide

1. The structure that does most of the work of inhalation in quiet breathing

          _____

2. The gas that yields bicarbonate ions when it dissolves in the blood

          _____

3. The space between the two vocal cords

          _____

4. The small air sacs in the lungs through which gases are exchanged

          _____

5. The serous membrane around each lung

          _____

6. An enzyme in red blood cells that speeds the production of bicarbonate ion in the blood

          _____

7. The space between the lungs in which the heart and other structures are located

          _____

8. The smallest division of a bronchus

          _____

9. The substance that carries most of the oxygen in the blood

          _____

Group E

hypoxia   tracheostomy   pneumonectomy
thoracentesis   asthma   cardiopulmonary resuscitation
tracheotomy   emphysema   bronchoscope

1. Spasms of the bronchi and breathing difficulties associated with severe allergies

          _____

2. A lower than normal concentration of oxygen in the tissues _____

3. An operation to insert a metal or plastic tube into the trachea to serve as an airway for ventilation _____

4. An instrument used to inspect the bronchi and their branches _____

5. Complete surgical removal of a lung _____

6. Destruction of the alveoli of the lungs often related to heavy smoking _____

7. An incision into the trachea for the purpose of removing a foreign object or a growth _____

8. A first aid technique used to revive a person experiencing both respiratory and cardiac arrest _____

9. Insertion of a needle into the pleural space to remove fluid _____

Group F

tachypnea   atelectasis   dyspnea
elasticity   acute coryza   orthopnea
cyanosis   chemoreceptors   hypoventilation

1. The symptom of difficult or labored breathing _____

2. Incomplete expansion of a lung or part of a lung _____

3. The property that allows the lung and chest wall to recoil during exhalation _____

4. Condition in which an insufficient amount of air reaches the alveoli as a result, for example, of disease, injury, or respiratory obstruction _____

5. A bluish color of the skin and mucous membranes caused by an insufficient amount of oxygen in the blood _____

6. An excessive rate of breathing _____

7. Areas in the major arteries of the chest and neck that regulate breathing according to changes in the composition of the blood _____

8. Technical name for the common cold, based on the discharge of fluid from the nose _____

9. Difficulty in breathing that is relieved by an upright position _____

IV. Multiple Choice

Select the best answer and write the letter of your choice in the blank.

1. In respiration, gases move across epithelial membranes   1. _____
   by the process of

   a. filtration
   b. diffusion
   c. active transport
   d. carriers
   e. phagocytosis

2. Which of the following terms does *not* apply to the cells that   2. _____
   line the conducting passages of the respiratory tract?

   a. ciliated
   b. pseudostratified
   c. epithelial
   d. pleural
   e. columnar

3. A structural defect of the partition in the nose is called a(n)   3. _____

   a. deviated septum
   b. pleural adhesion
   c. polyp
   d. epistaxis
   e. bifurcation

4. The bones that form the nasal septum are the   4. _____

   a. frontal and parietal
   b. ethmoid and vomer
   c. temporal and lacrimal
   d. nasal and maxilla
   e. ethmoid and sphenoid

5. The respiratory control centers are located in the parts of the   5. _____
   brain stem called the

   a. cortex and spinal cord
   b. medulla and midbrain
   c. thalamus and pons
   d. pineal and ventricle
   e. pons and medulla

6. A rhythmic abnormality in breathing that is seen in critically   6. _____
   ill patients is termed

   a. hypoxemia
   b. hyperpnea
   c. Cheyne-Stokes respiration
   d. effusion
   e. hyaline membrane disease

7. Allergic rhinitis is the medical term for   7. _____

   a. hives
   b. nosebleed
   c. hay fever
   d. cancer
   e. adhesion

8. An average total lung capacity is   8. _____

   a. 6000 mL
   b. 500 mL
   c. 60 L
   d. 2400 mL
   e. 6000 g

9. The functional residual capacity is   9. _____

   a. the amount of air that can be moved into or out of the
      lungs after surgery
   b. the amount of air that is always in the lungs
   c. all of the air in the lungs except the residual volume
   d. the amount of air in the lungs after normal exhalation
   e. the amount of air that can be forced out of the lungs

10. Hemothorax is the   10. _____

   a. presence of air in the pleural space
   b. presence of pus in the pleural space
   c. removal of air from the pleural space
   d. presence of blood in the pleural space
   e. removal of fluid from the pleural space

V. Labeling

For each of the following illustrations, write the name or names of each labeled part on the numbered lines.

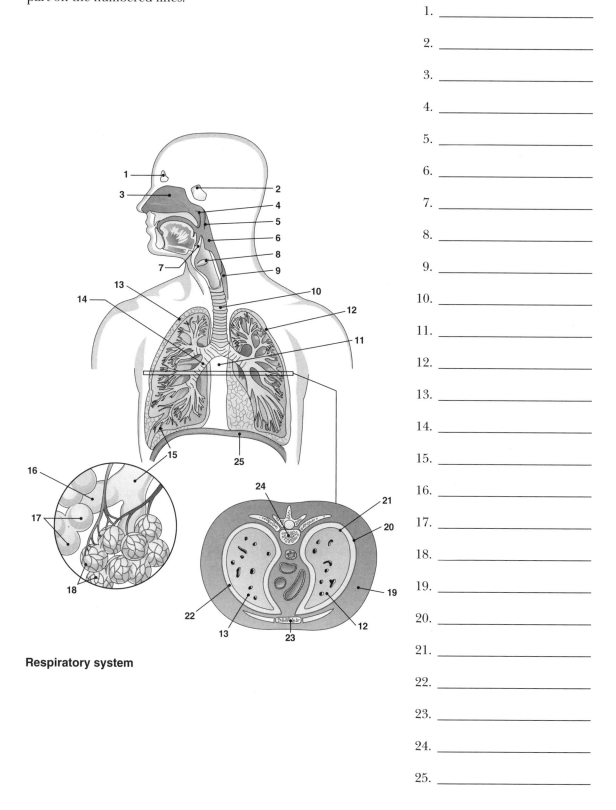

Respiratory system

1. _____

2. _____

3. _____

4. _____

5. _____

6. _____

7. _____

8. _____

9. _____

10. _____

11. _____

12. _____

13. _____

14. _____

15. _____

16. _____

17. _____

18. _____

19. _____

20. _____

21. _____

22. _____

23. _____

24. _____

25. _____

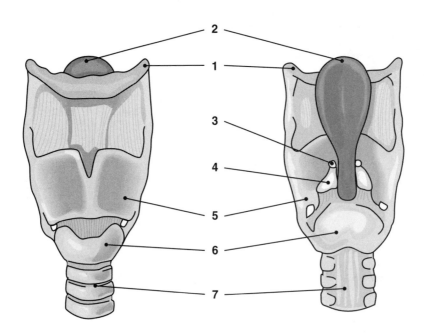

The larynx

1. _____   5. _____

2. _____   6. _____

3. _____   7. _____

4. _____

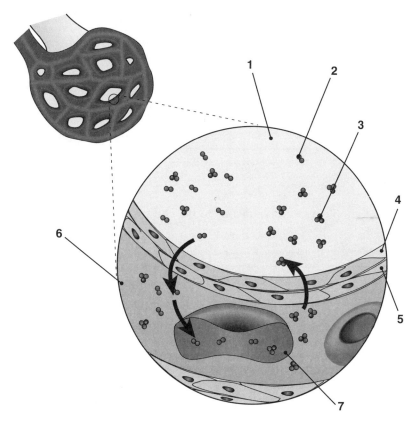

Diffusion of gas molecules in the lungs

1. _____   5. _____

2. _____   6. _____

3. _____   7. _____

4. _____

VI. True–False

For each question, write T for true or F for false in the blank to the left of each number. If a statement is false, correct it by replacing the underlined term and write the correct statement in the blanks below the question.

_____ 1. The left bronchus divides into <u>two</u> secondary bronchi.

_____

_____

_____ 2. The portion of the pleura that is attached to the chest wall is the <u>parietal</u> pleura.

_____

_____

_____ 3. The wall of an alveolus is made of <u>stratified</u> squamous epithelium.

_____

_____

_____ 4. The phrenic nerve stimulates the <u>lungs</u>.

_____

_____

_____ 5. The passive phase of relaxed breathing is <u>exhalation</u>.

_____

_____

_____ 6. As carbon dioxide levels increase, the blood becomes more <u>alkaline</u>.

_____

_____

_____ 7. The form of pneumonia in which the disease is scattered through the lung is <u>bronchopneumonia</u>.

_____

_____

_____ 8. A temporary cessation of breathing, as may occur during sleep, is hyperpnea.

_____

_____

_____ 9. The amount of air that remains in the lung after maximum exhalation is the total lung capacity.

_____

_____

_____ 10. Hyperventilation results in an increase of carbon dioxide in the blood.

_____

_____

VII. Completion Exercise

Write the word or phrase that correctly completes each sentence.

1. A lower than normal level of oxygen in arterial blood is called _____

2. The substance in red blood cells that transports oxygen is _____

3. Heart disease and other disorders may cause the bluish color of the skin and visible mucous membranes characteristic of a condition called _____

4. An injury or a blow to the nose is a frequent cause of nosebleed, or _____

5. The volume of air that can be expelled from the lungs by maximum exhalation after maximum inhalation is the _____

6. In COPD, there is damage to the small airways and poor exchange of gases. A symptom of this disorder is difficult or labored breathing called _____

7. An abnormal increase in the depth and rate of respiration is termed _____

8. Inflammation of the membranes around the lungs is called _____

9. The organism that causes tuberculosis is named _____

10. Certain diplococci, staphylococci, chlamydias, and viruses may cause an inflammation of the lungs. The disease is called _____

11. The term that is used for the pressure of each gas in a mixture of gases is _____

VIII. Practical Applications

Study each discussion. Then write the appropriate word or phrase in the space provided.

Group A

1. Mrs. D brought her toddler Caren into the pediatrician's office because the child had a runny nose, slight fever, and was irritable. The physician prescribed medication to relieve the symptoms and instructed Mrs. D to call if the child developed additional signs, such as high fever or rash, that might indicate more serious illness. The diagnosis the physician wrote on Caren's medical record was abbreviated URI, which stands for _____

2. G, age 14, complained of a sore throat and difficulty in swallowing. Using the scientific name for the throat, the physician described the disorder as _____

3. Ms. F, age 34, complained of hoarseness and said that it was causing her difficulty in speaking to her students. This inflammation of the larynx is called _____

4. Mrs. L had been suffering from a cold for several days. The physician explained that no entirely effective method for preventing the common cold is known as yet. The cause of colds is a group of highly variable and contagious agents classified as _____

5. Because of Mrs. L's lowered disease resistance, she was also suffering from inflammation of the bronchi and their subdivisions. This infection is called _____

6. The physician warned Mrs. L that if she did not stop working temporarily and get sufficient rest to increase her disease resistance, her illness might extend into the lung, an infection known as _____

7. Mr. M, age 47, was advised to see his physician because a routine x-ray examination performed at his place of work revealed a lung lesion. Mr. M was a chain smoker. The possibility of a malignancy of the type that originates in a bronchus was being considered. This most common form of lung cancer is _____

Group B

1. Teenage Jim was brought to the hospital after an automobile accident. There were signs of chest injury, and he was having great difficulty breathing. It was probable that there was air in the pleural space, a condition called _____

2. As a result of tuberculosis, Mrs. S, age 67, suffered from a painful condition that involved inflammation and adhesion of the membranes around the lungs. Inflammation of these membranes is termed _____

3. Mrs. S's complaints included shortness of breath, a chronic cough productive of thick mucus, and a "chest cold" of 2 months' duration. She was advised to quit smoking, a major cause of lung irritation in a group of chronic lung diseases collectively known as

_____

4. Symptoms in Mrs. S's case were due in part to the obstruction of groups of alveoli by mucous plugs. A chest film showed patches of collapsed alveoli, a condition that the radiologist identified as

_____

5. Evaluation of Mrs. S's respiratory function showed reduction in the amount of air that could be moved into and out of her lungs. The amount of air that can be expelled by maximum exhalation following maximum inhalation is termed the

_____

6. Allison, a student trying out for high-school drill team, felt nervous about her performance. She was observed to have alternating episodes of apnea and rapid breathing, a common response of the respiratory center to abnormal levels of carbon dioxide produced by

_____

IX. Short Essays

1. Compare the terms *respiration* and *cellular respiration*.

_____

_____

_____

2. Name some parts of the respiratory tract where gas exchange does *not* occur.

_____

_____

_____

3. Explain the role of chemoreceptors in the control of respiration.

_____

_____

_____

19

Digestion

I. Overview

The food we eat is made available to cells throughout the body by the complex processes of *digestion* and *absorption*. These are the functions of the *digestive system*, composed of the *digestive tract* and the *accessory organs*.

The digestive tract, consisting of the *mouth*, the *pharynx*, the *esophagus*, the *stomach*, and the small and large *intestine*, forms a continuous passageway in which ingested food is prepared for use by the body and waste products are collected to be expelled from the body. The accessory organs, the *salivary glands*, *liver*, *gallbladder*, and *pancreas*, manufacture various enzymes and other substances needed in digestion. They also serve as storage areas for substances that are released as required.

Digestion begins in the mouth with the digestion of starch. It continues in the stomach, where proteins are digested, and is completed in the small intestine. Most absorption of digested food also occurs in the small intestine through small projections of the lining called *villi.*

The process of digestion is controlled by both nervous and hormonal mechanisms, which regulate the activity of the digestive organs and the rate at which food moves through the digestive tract.

II. Topics for Review

A. Wall of the digestive tract
B. The peritoneum
C. Organs of the digestive tract and their functions
D. Accessory organs and their functions
E. The process of digestion

1. Enzymes
2. Water
3. Other substances
F. Absorption
G. Control of the digestive process
    1. Nervous
    2. Hormonal
H. Disorders of the digestive system

III. Matching Exercises

Matching only within each group, write the answers in the spaces provided.

Group A

deciduous   absorption   mastication
digestion   ingestion   peristalsis
peritoneum   secretin

1. The process by which food is converted into substances
   small enough to be taken into the cells _____

2. Term that describes the baby teeth, based on the fact
   that they are lost _____

3. The transfer of digested food into the bloodstream _____

4. A hormone that stimulates digestion _____

5. The rhythmic motion that propels food along the digestive tract

_____

6. The process of chewing

_____

7. The intake of food into the digestive tract

_____

8. The largest serous membrane in the body

_____

Group B

premolars   parotid   uvula
caries   canines   incisors
molars   submandibular

1. The scientific name for tooth decay

_____

2. Name of the salivary glands that are located near the body of the lower jaw

_____

3. The eight cutting teeth located in the front part of the oral cavity

_____

4. Another name for the eye teeth

_____

5. The permanent teeth that replace the baby molars; the bicuspids

_____

6. A fleshy mass that hangs from the soft palate

_____

7. The largest of the salivary glands

_____

8. The grinding teeth located in the back part of the oral cavity

_____

Group C

sphincter   esophagus   deglutition
amylase   gingivitis   pharynx
parotitis   periodontitis

1. The scientific name for the throat

_____

2. The act of swallowing

_____

3. Infection of the gums

_____

4. A circular muscle that acts as a valve

_____

5. The enzyme in saliva that digests starch

_____

6. The tube that carries food into the stomach

_____

7. The medical name for mumps

_____

8. Infection of the gums and the bones supporting the teeth _____

Group D

cholecystokinin	greater omentum	rugae
mesocolon	villi	mesentery
parietal	anus	submucosa

1. The distal opening of the digestive tract _____

2. The numerous tiny projections in the small intestine that greatly increase its absorbing surface _____

3. A hormone that stimulates digestion _____

4. Term that describes the layer of a serous membrane that lines a body cavity _____

5. The layer of connective tissue beneath the mucous membrane in the wall of the digestive tract _____

6. The double-layered portion of the peritoneum that is attached to the small intestine _____

7. Folds that appear in the lining of the stomach when it is empty _____

8. The section of the peritoneum that extends from the colon to the back wall of the abdomen _____

9. An apronlike double membrane that extends downward from the stomach _____

Group E

lower esophageal sphincter	flatulence	vomiting
bolus	soft palate	epiglottis
chyme	pyloric sphincter	

1. The mixture that forms in the stomach when food is combined with gastric juice _____

2. A condition that results from accumulation of excessive air (gas) in the stomach or intestine _____

3. The valve between the distal end of the stomach and the small intestine _____

4. The back portion of the oral cavity roof _____

5. The structure that guards the entrance into the stomach _____

6. A structure that covers the opening of the larynx during swallowing _____

7. Reverse peristalsis that forces gastric contents through the mouth

_____

8. A small portion of food mixed with saliva that is pushed into the pharynx in swallowing

_____

Group F

ascites   gastric ulcer   ileocecal valve
jejunum   ileum   duodenum
hemorrhoids   hepatitis   adenocarcinoma

1. The second part of the small intestine

_____

2. The sphincter between the small and large intestine

_____

3. The most frequent type of stomach cancer, which originates in the stomach lining

_____

4. The final, and longest, section of the small intestine

_____

5. Inflammation of the liver

_____

6. The accumulation of fluid in the peritoneal cavity, as may occur in certain serious illnesses

_____

7. Enlargement of the veins in the rectum

_____

8. The first part of the small intestine

_____

9. An area of destruction of the mucous membrane lining the stomach

_____

Group G

fats   trypsin   lipase
starch   albumin   urea
carbohydrates   proteins   glycogen

1. The form in which glucose is stored in the liver

_____

2. A plasma protein produced in the liver

_____

3. The type of food that is digested by bile

_____

4. A class of organic chemicals that includes sugars and starches

_____

5. The waste product manufactured in the liver that is later eliminated by the kidneys

_____

6. The type of food that is digested by gastric juice

_____

7. An enzyme that breaks fats into simpler compounds in digestion

_____

8. The nutrient that is digested by pancreatic amylase

    _____

9. A pancreatic enzyme that splits proteins into amino acids

    _____

Group H

hydrolysis	colon	feces
cecum	gallbladder	small intestine
pepsin	liver	lacteals

1. The enzyme that digests proteins in the stomach

    _____

2. The major portion of the large intestine

    _____

3. The organ from which most digested food is absorbed into the bloodstream

    _____

4. The splitting of food molecules by the addition of water

    _____

5. The small pouch at the beginning of the large intestine

    _____

6. The solid waste products of digestion

    _____

7. The lymphatic capillaries in the villi of the small intestine that absorb digested fats

    _____

8. An organ that stores nutrients and releases them as needed into the bloodstream

    _____

9. The accessory organ that stores bile

    _____

Group I

vermiform appendix	rectum	cholecystitis
gastroenteritis	jaundice	defecation
colonoscope	cirrhosis	diverticula

1. A type of liver damage commonly caused by alcohol abuse

    _____

2. An instrument used to examine the large intestine

    _____

3. Inflammation of the stomach and intestine

    _____

4. Abnormal saclike bulges in the intestinal wall

    _____

5. The part of the large intestine between the sigmoid colon and the anus

    _____

6. Elimination of the stool

    _____

7. The small blind tube attached to the cecum

    _____

8. Inflammation of the gallbladder

    _____

9. A yellow coloration of the skin caused by accumulation
   of bile pigments in the blood
   _____

IV. Multiple Choice

Select the best answer and write the letter of your choice in the blank.

1. Which of the following is *not* a portion of the peritoneum?   1. _____

   a. mesocolon
   b. lesser omentum
   c. mesentery
   d. hiatus
   e. greater omentum

2. A highly contagious type of gingivitis due to a spirochete or a   2. _____
   bacillus that is characterized by inflammation and ulceration is called

   a. Vincent's disease
   b. peritonitis
   c. cirrhosis
   d. enteritis
   e. leukoplakia

3. Which of the following is *not* associated with the accessory   3. _____
   organs of digestion?

   a. salivary glands
   b. vermiform appendix
   c. cystic duct
   d. pancreas
   e. common bile duct

4. The adjective *hepatic* refers to the   4. _____

   a. spleen
   b. liver
   c. gallbladder
   d. ileum
   e. duodenum

5. The active ingredients in gastric juice are   5. _____

   a. bile and trypsin
   b. amylase and pepsin
   c. pepsin and hydrochloric acid
   d. maltase and secretin
   e. sodium bicarbonate and GIP

6. An instrument used to examine the lower portion of the colon is a(n)   6. _____

   a. sigmoidoscope
   b. bronchoscope
   c. electroencephalogram
   d. culposcope
   e. electrocardiogram

7. Which of the following is *not* associated with the stomach?   7. _____

   a. greater curvature
   b. rugae
   c. lacteals
   d. pylorus
   e. LES

8. The sublingual salivary glands are located   8. _____

   a. on the tongue
   b. under the tongue
   c. in the cheek
   d. in the oropharynx
   e. in front of the uvula

9. Which of the following does *not* occur in the mouth?   9. _____

   a. ingestion
   b. mastication
   c. moistening of food
   d. digestion of starch
   e. absorption of nutrients

10. Which of the following is the correct order of tissue from the   10. _____
    innermost to the outermost layer in the wall of the digestive tract?

    a. smooth muscle, serous membrane, mucous membrane, submucosa
    b. submucosa, serous membrane, smooth muscle, mucous membrane
    c. serous membrane, smooth muscle, submucosa, mucosa
    d. mucous membrane, submucosa, smooth muscle, serous membrane
    e. none of the above

11. Which of the following is *not* a hormone used in digestion?   11. _____

    a. CCK
    b. GIP
    c. secretin
    d. nuclease
    e. gastrin

12. Crohn's disease is   12. _____

    a. ulceration of the stomach
    b. inflammation of the uvula
    c. flaccid constipation
    d. inflammation of the peritoneal cavity
    e. an inflammatory disease of the intestine

V. Labeling

For each of the following illustrations, write the name or names of each labeled part on the numbered lines.

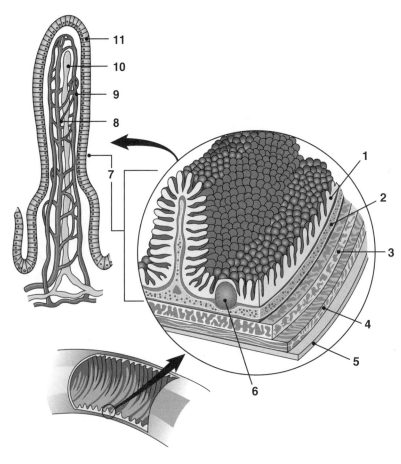

Wall of the small intestine

1. _____

2. _____

3. _____

4. _____

5. _____

6. _____

7. _____

8. _____

9. _____

10. _____

11. _____

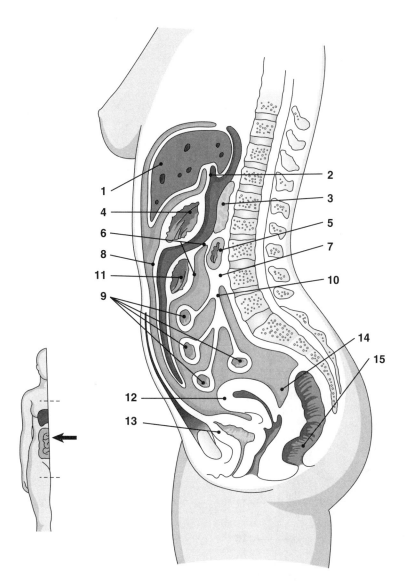

Abdominal cavity showing peritoneum

1. _____

2. _____

3. _____

4. _____

5. _____

6. _____

7. _____

8. _____

9. _____

10. _____

11. _____

12. _____

13. _____

14. _____

15. _____

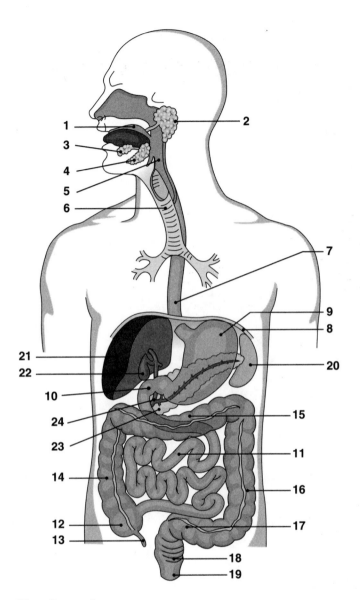

Digestive system

1. _____
2. _____
3. _____
4. _____
5. _____
6. _____
7. _____
8. _____
9. _____
10. _____
11. _____
12. _____
13. _____
14. _____
15. _____
16. _____
17. _____
18. _____
19. _____
20. _____
21. _____
22. _____
23. _____
24. _____

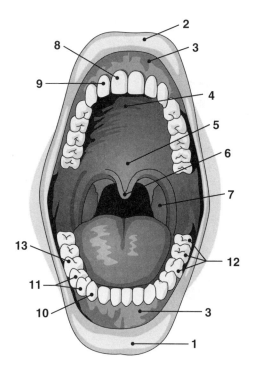

The mouth

1. _____

2. _____

3. _____

4. _____

5. _____

6. _____

7. _____

8. _____

9. _____

10. _____

11. _____

12. _____

13. _____

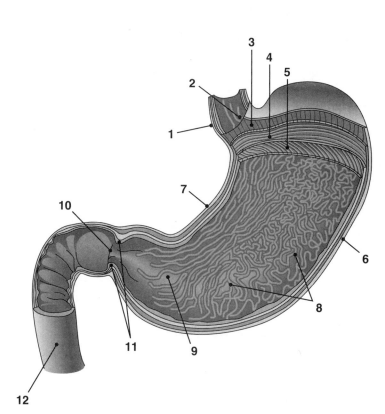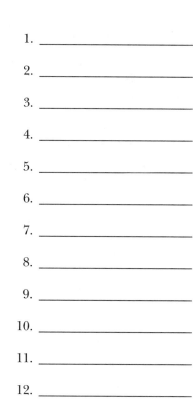

Longitudinal section of the stomach

1. _____

2. _____

3. _____

4. _____

5. _____

6. _____

7. _____

8. _____

9. _____

10. _____

11. _____

12. _____

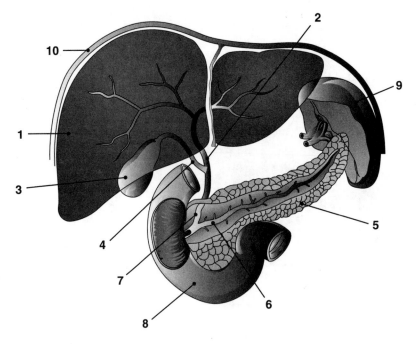

Accessory organs of digestion

1. _____   6. _____

2. _____   7. _____

3. _____   8. _____

4. _____   9. _____

5. _____   10. _____

VI. True–False

For each question, write T for true or F for false in the blank to the left of each number. If a statement is false, correct it by replacing the <u>underlined</u> term and write the correct statement in the blanks below the question.

_____ 1. There are <u>32</u> deciduous teeth.

_____

_____

_____ 2. Most digested fats are absorbed into the <u>lymph.</u>

_____

_____

_____ 3. The part of the peritoneum that is attached to the small intestine is the <u>mesocolon.</u>

_____

_____

_____ 4. The lower esophageal sphincter is also called the <u>pyloric sphincter.</u>

_____

_____

_____ 5. The <u>greater omentum</u> extends between the stomach and the liver.

_____

_____

_____ 6. The <u>jejunum</u> is the middle portion of the small intestine.

_____

_____

_____ 7. The descending colon is located in the <u>left portion</u> of the abdomen.

_____

_____

_____ 8. The common hepatic duct and the cystic duct merge to form the <u>common bile duct.</u>

_____

_____

_____ 9. The cystic duct drains bile from the <u>gallbladder.</u>

_____

_____

_____ 10. Gastrin is a hormone that stimulates the <u>pancreas.</u>

_____

_____

_____ 11. Monosaccharides are the building blocks of <u>carbohydrates.</u>

_____

_____

_____ 12. In <u>spastic</u> constipation, the intestinal muscle is atonic.

_____

_____

_____ 13. Lipases are enzymes that digest <u>fats.</u>

_____

_____

VII. Completion Exercise

Write the word or phrase that correctly completes each sentence.

1. The serous membrane that lines the abdominal cavity and covers the abdominal organs is the

_____

2. A common cause of tooth loss is infection of the gums and bone around the teeth, a condition called

_____

3. Saliva is produced by three pairs of glands, of which the largest are the ones located near the angles of the jaw. These are the

_____

4. Such symptoms as nausea, vomiting, diarrhea, and severe abdominal pain are characteristic of an inflammation that involves the stomach and small intestine. This disorder is called

_____

5. Examination of the interior of an organ with a flexible tube is called

_____

6. Any inflammation of the liver is called

_____

7. Most of the digestive juices contain substances that cause the chemical breakdown of foods without entering into the reaction themselves. These catalytic agents are

_____

8. One component of gastric juice kills bacteria and thus helps defend the body against disease. This substance is

_____

9. Starches and sugars are classified as _____

10. One inflammatory condition in which the pancreas is actually destroyed by the juice it produces is called _____

11. The lower part of the colon bends into an S shape, so this part is called the _____

12. A temporary storage section for indigestible and unabsorbable waste products of digestion is a tube called the _____

13. The distal portion of the large intestine leads to the outside through an opening called the _____

14. The muscular sac in which bile is stored to be released as needed is called the _____

15. A disorder characterized by abdominal pain and alternating episodes of constipation and diarrhea is called _____

VIII. Practical Applications

Study each discussion. Then write the appropriate word or phrase in the space provided.

1. Mr. C, age 36, was a tense man who divided up his long working hours with coffee and cigarette breaks. After work, he would frequently consume alcoholic beverages before dinner. Endoscopy showed inflammation of the lining of the stomach. The name of the innermost layer of the stomach is _____

2. Mr. C also complained of pain in the "pit of the stomach." Until recently, eating seemed to provide some relief. The endoscopy also showed a damaged area located in the first part of the small intestine. This section of the small intestine is called the _____

3. Three-month-old John was brought to the clinic by his mother because he had suffered several bouts of vomiting and could not retain food. The tentative diagnosis was a constricted and obstructive pyloric sphincter, a condition called _____

4. Mrs. K, age 24, complained that since returning from a brief trip out of the United States she was suffering from frequent watery stools. This symptom is called _____

5. Mrs. D, age 41, complained of indigestion, belching, and abdominal pain. The pain in the upper right side of the abdomen and right shoulder became so severe that she reported to the emergency room. She was diagnosed as having a disorder involving stones in the gallbladder, a condition that is referred to medically as _____

6. Mr. B had suffered acute abdominal pain and other symptoms of appendicitis. Because of his delay in seeking treatment, his appendix ruptured. He required exacting care following surgery because of a serious infection of the abdominal serosa. This disorder is called _____

7. After a long delay, Mr. C reported to the doctor's office with a request from his dentist that a number of white patches in his mouth undergo further testing. A biopsy was performed, with a diagnosis of cancer of the mouth. These white patches characterize a condition that is common in smokers and may lead to cancer, a condition that is called _____

8. Mr. J, age 42, was admitted to the hospital after a 3-day drinking binge. He had severe epigastric pain, jaundice, fever, and vomiting. On physical examination, the edge of the liver was felt 5 cm (2 in) below the ribs. A biopsy of the liver indicated chronic alcoholic cirrhosis. The jaundice associated with this condition results from the release of a hepatic secretion into the bloodstream. This secretion, which is needed in digestion, is named _____

9. Mrs. L complained of discomfort in the upper region of the abdomen after eating. Her physician ordered a radiographic study of the upper GI tract. She suspected a weakness in the diaphragm where the esophagus passes through. This weakness can allow the stomach to protrude through the diaphragm, a condition known as _____

IX. Short Essays

1. Briefly explain how the process of digestion is regulated.

_____

_____

_____

2. The hepatic portal system carries blood from the digestive organs to the liver. Explain why this is necessary.

_____

_____

_____

3. Describe some features of the small intestine that increase the surface area for absorption of nutrients.

_____

_____

_____

20

Metabolism, Nutrition, and Body Temperature

I. Overview

The nutrients that reach the cells following digestion and absorption are used to maintain life. All the physical and chemical reactions that occur within the cells make up *metabolism,* which has two phases: a breakdown phase, or *catabolism,* and a building phase, or *anabolism.* In catabolism, nutrients are oxidized to yield energy for the cells in the form of ATP. This process, termed *cellular respiration,* occurs in two steps: the first is anaerobic (does not require oxygen) and produces a small amount of energy; the second is aerobic (requires oxygen). This second step occurs within the mitochondria of the cells. It yields a large amount of the energy contained in the nutrient plus carbon dioxide and water.

By the various pathways of metabolism, the breakdown products of food can be built into substances needed by the body. The *essential* amino acids and fatty acids cannot be manufactured internally and must be taken in with the diet. Minerals and vitamins are also needed in the diet for health. Because ingested food is the source of all nourishment for the body, a balanced diet should be followed and "food fads" should be avoided.

The rate at which energy is released from nutrients is termed the *metabolic rate.* It is affected by many factors including age, size, sex, activity, and hormones. Some of the energy in nutrients is released in the form of heat, which serves to maintain body temperature. A steady temperature of about 37°C (98.6°F) is maintained by several mechanisms.

Heat production is greatly increased during periods of increased muscular or glandular activity. Most heat loss occurs through the skin, with a smaller loss by way of the respiratory system and the urine and feces. The *hypothalamus* of the brain maintains the normal temperature in response to the temperature of the blood and information received from temperature receptors in the skin. Regulation occurs through vasodilation and vasoconstriction of the surface blood vessels, activity of the sweat glands, and muscle activity.

Abnormalities of body temperature are a valuable diagnostic tool. The presence of *fever*—an abnormally high body temperature—usually indicates infection, but may also indicate a toxic reaction, a brain injury, and other disorders. The opposite of fever is *hypothermia*—an exceedingly low body temperature—which most often occurs when the body is exposed to very low outside temperature. Hypothermia can cause serious damage to the body tissues.

II. Topics for Review

A. Metabolism
 1. Catabolism and anabolism
 2. Cellular respiration
 3. Metabolic rate
B. Use of nutrients
 1. Essential amino acids and fatty acids
 2. Minerals and vitamins
C. Nutrition guidelines
 1. Carbohydrates, fats, and proteins
 2. Supplements
 3. Alcohol

D. Body temperature
   1. Heat production
   2. Heat loss
   3. Temperature regulation
      a. Role of the hypothalamus
   4. Normal and abnormal body temperature

III. Matching Exercises

Matching only within each group, write the answers in the spaces provided.

Group A

anabolism	kilocalorie	catabolism
mitochondria	glycogen	anaerobic
amino acid	ATP	

1. The storage form of glucose   _____

2. The metabolic building of simple compounds into
   substances needed by cells   _____

3. Term that describes the first phase of cellular respiration
   because it does not require oxygen   _____

4. The unit used to measure the energy in foods   _____

5. A building block of proteins   _____

6. The metabolic breakdown of complex compounds   _____

7. The cell organelles in which the aerobic steps of
   metabolism occur   _____

8. A compound that stores energy in the cell   _____

Group B

glucose	minerals	enzymes
oxidation	glycerol	saturated
essential	allergy	

1. A component of fats   _____

2. The nutrient that is the main energy source for cells   _____

3. The catalysts of metabolic reactions   _____

4. The chemical term for the breakdown of nutrients to
   release energy   _____

5. An adverse immunologic reaction caused by certain
   foods in some people   _____

6. Term for fats that commonly are from animal sources and are solid at room temperature

_____

7. Term for an amino acid that must be taken in as part of the diet

_____

8. Elements needed for proper nutrition

_____

Group C

niacin	calciferol	iron
vitamin B_1	vitamin A	vitamin B_{12}
vitamin C	folate	calcium

1. Another name for vitamin D, the vitamin required for normal bone formation

_____

2. The characteristic element in hemoglobin, the oxygen-carrying compound in the blood

_____

3. The vitamin that prevents dry, scaly skin and night blindness

_____

4. The vitamin needed to prevent anemia, digestive disorders, and neural tube defects in the embryo

_____

5. A mineral needed for proper bone development that is found in dairy products and vegetables

_____

6. Another name for thiamin, a deficiency of which will result in beriberi

_____

7. The vitamin found in yeast, meat, grains, nuts, and legumes and needed to prevent pellagra

_____

8. The vitamin that is also called ascorbic acid

_____

9. The vitamin needed for blood cell formation that is found in meat, milk, and eggs

_____

Group D

conduction	hypothermia	febrile
homeostasis	cellular respiration	insulation
hypothalamus	circulation	

1. The chief heat-regulating center, located in the brain

_____

2. A series of metabolic reactions in which energy is released from nutrients; also described as oxidation

_____

3. The transfer of heat to the surrounding air _____

4. The tendency of body processes to maintain a constant state _____

5. An abnormally low temperature, as may be caused by prolonged exposure to cold _____

6. The term that describes a person who has a fever _____

7. Prevention of heat loss _____

8. A means for distributing heat throughout the body _____

Group E

crisis	constriction	phagocytosis
heat stroke	evaporation	lysis
heat exhaustion	infection	

1. A sudden drop in temperature at the end of a period of fever _____

2. The change that occurs in blood vessels of the skin if too much heat is being lost from the body _____

3. A condition that may follow heat cramps if adequate treatment is not given _____

4. Heat loss resulting from the conversion of a liquid, such as perspiration, to a vapor _____

5. A process by which leukocytes destroy pathogens _____

6. A gradual fall in temperature at the end of a period of fever _____

7. A common cause of fever _____

8. The final stages of excessive exposure to heat, characterized by central nervous system symptoms _____

IV. Multiple Choice

Select the best answer and write the letter of your choice in the blank.

1. The amount of energy needed to maintain life functions while the body is at rest is

    1. _____

    a. basal metabolism
    b. metabolic rate
    c. anabolic rate
    d. rate of conduction
    e. hyperthermia

2. Glycogen is stored in the

    a. blood vessels and nerves
    b. heart and brain
    c. kidney and spleen
    d. bones and fat
    e. liver and muscles

2. _____

3. Peas and beans are classified as

    a. minerals
    b. grains
    c. cereals
    d. legumes
    e. lipids

3. _____

4. A complete protein has

    a. all the amino acids
    b. all the essential fatty acids
    c. a variety of vitamins
    d. all the essential amino acids
    e. a variety of minerals

4. _____

5. The end product of the anaerobic phase of glucose metabolism is

    a. glycogen
    b. pyruvic acid
    c. folic acid
    d. tocopherol
    e. chromium

5. _____

6. An element required for fluid balance and normal activity of nerves and muscles and that is found in fruits, meats, seafood, milk, and vegetables is

    a. glycerol
    b. potassium
    c. copper
    d. niacin
    e. pyridoxine

6. _____

7. Deamination is the

    a. conversion of glucose into glycogen
    b. building of amino acids into protein
    c. reduction of fever
    d. the first step in metabolism of alcohol
    e. removal of a nitrogen group from an amino acid

7. _____

8. Trace elements in the diet are   8. _____

   a. nonessential elements
   b. vitamins needed in very small amounts
   c. minerals needed in large quantity
   d. minerals needed in very small amounts
   e. organic elements

9. The largest amount of heat is produced in the body by   9. _____

   a. muscles and glands
   b. cartilage and adipose tissue
   c. epithelium and blood
   d. nerves and tendons
   e. sense organs and lymphoid tissue

10. A pyrogen is a(n)   10. _____

    a. vitamin
    b. substance that produces convection
    c. substance that produces fever
    d. antipyretic
    e. substance that causes lysis

11. Which of the following is *not* an avenue for heat loss   11. _____
    from the body?

    a. feces
    b. skin
    c. muscles
    d. expired air
    e. urine

V. True–False

For each question, write T for true or F for false in the blank to the left of each
number. If a statement is false, correct it by replacing the underlined term and
write the correct statement in the blanks below the question.

_____ 1. An aerobic reaction requires <u>oxygen.</u>

_____

_____

_____ 2. The anaerobic phase of cellular respiration yields <u>34 to 36</u> ATP per
           glucose.

_____

_____

_____ 3. The building phase of metabolism is called <u>catabolism.</u>

_____

_____

_____ 4. There are <u>nine</u> essential amino acids.

_____

_____

_____ 5. The B vitamins are <u>fat</u> soluble.

_____

_____

_____ 6. Most heat loss in the body occurs through the <u>skin.</u>

_____

_____

_____ 7. The element nitrogen is found in all <u>proteins.</u>

_____

_____

_____ 8. Alcohol yields <u>7 kcal</u> per gram.

_____

_____

_____ 9. It is recommended that more than half of the calories in the diet should come from <u>fats.</u>

_____

_____

_____ 10. Most oils are <u>unsaturated</u> fats.

_____

_____

_____ 11. <u>Water-soluble</u> vitamins are not stored in the body.

_____

_____

_____ 12. When body temperature rises above normal, the blood vessels <u>constrict.</u>

_____

_____

_____ 13. A fan increases heat loss by the process of <u>convection.</u>

_____

_____

VI. Completion Exercise

Write the word or phrase that correctly completes each sentence.

1. All the chemical reactions that sustain life together make up

    _____

2. Organic substances needed in small amounts in the diet are the

    _____

3. A gland important in the control of the metabolic rate is the

    _____

4. The most important heat-regulating center is a section of the brain called the

    _____

5. Shivering is a way of increasing body heat by increasing the activity of the

    _____

6. During a fever, there may be considerable destruction of body tissues. Therefore, the diet should include nitrogen-containing foods classified as

    _____

7. Tissue damage caused by exposure to cold is termed

    _____

8. The normal range of body temperature in degrees Celsius is

    _____

9. The formula for converting Fahrenheit temperatures to Celsius is

_____

10. Practice changing Fahrenheit to Celsius. Show the figures for changing 50°F and 70°F to Celsius.

_____

11. Practice changing Celsius to Fahrenheit. Show the figures for changing 10°C and 25°C to Fahrenheit.

_____

VII. Practical Applications

Study each discussion. Then write the appropriate word or phrase in the space provided.

Group A

1. Mrs. S, age 76, was scheduled to have the bones in her fractured femur pinned. The radiographs taken after her fall showed that her bones lacked density, as if there were insufficient deposit of a mineral needed for bone strength. This mineral is also needed for blood clotting, muscle contractions, and nerve impulse conduction. The mineral is

_____

2. Mr. C, age 78, was accompanied by his daughter to visit his family physician. His daughter was concerned about his general state of health and marked weight loss within several months after the death of his wife. The doctor asked that Mr. C keep a record of his food intake for 2 weeks. Review of this record suggested that he was not eating properly and was suffering from a general lack of proper nutrients in his diet. The doctor described his condition as one of borderline

_____

3. Young Mr. N, age 17, had placed himself on a strict vegetarian diet that included no animal products. He was not careful in planning his meals, however, and his family soon began to notice his loss of appetite, irritability, and susceptibility to disease. The school dietitian, when questioned by his mother, suggested that he was not getting the right balance of proteins, especially the building blocks of proteins that must be taken in with the diet, the

_____

4. When Ms. R, age 15, went for her regular dental examination, the dentist noticed that her gums bled easily and that she had small cracks at the corners of her mouth. Brief questioning suggested that because of a lack of fruits and vegetables in her diet she was suffering from a lack of vitamins, especially vitamin C and a group of vitamins that includes thiamin and riboflavin, the

_____

Group B

A physician working in a desert area of southeastern California saw a variety of cases during the course of a day.

1. A 6-year-old patient appeared apathetic and tired. His face was flushed and hot. On taking his temperature, the nurse found it to be 105°F. The physician took the child's history and examined him, then instructed his mother to give the child cool sponge baths and administer the prescribed medication. The cool water would draw heat from the body in changing from a liquid to a vapor, reducing body temperature by the process of _____

2. Men working on a construction project complained of tiredness, nausea, and a rapid pulse. They felt better after resting in the shade and drinking water and fruit juices. Their condition, caused by exposure to high outside temperatures, is clinically described as _____

3. Mr. K, age 69, was normally inactive. Today, he had spent all afternoon repairing a fence. His wife found him wandering aimlessly outside, noted that his skin was red, hot, and dry, and brought him to the doctor. His symptoms indicated a medical emergency known as _____

4. On a cool fall day, Mr. J spent several hours walking with friends in the canyons of some nearby mountains. He was clad in shorts and a lightweight shirt. Now, he was stumbling, his speech was difficult to understand, and he complained of being sleepy. He probably had a condition of low body temperature called _____

VIII. Short Essays

1. Compare saturated and unsaturated fats, giving examples of each type, and cite the significance of each in the diet.

_____

_____

_____

2. Compare water-soluble and fat-soluble vitamins and give examples of each.

_____

_____

_____

3. Explain briefly how body temperature is regulated.

_____

_____

_____

21

Body Fluids

I. Overview

From 50% to 70% of a person's body weight is water. This water serves as a solvent, a transport medium, and a participant in metabolic reactions. Dissolved in the water are a variety of substances, such as electrolytes, nutrients, gases, enzymes, hormones, and waste products. Body fluids are distributed in two main compartments:

1. The *intracellular fluid compartment* within the cells
2. The *extracellular fluid compartment* located outside the cells. This category includes blood plasma, interstitial fluid, lymph, and fluids in special compartments, such as the humors of the eye, cerebrospinal fluid, serous fluids, and synovial fluids.

Water balance is maintained by constant intake and output of fluids, as controlled by the thirst center in the hypothalamus. Normally, the amount of fluid taken in with food and beverages equals the amount of fluid lost through the skin and the respiratory, digestive, and urinary tracts. When there is an imbalance between fluid intake and fluid output, serious disorders such as edema, water intoxication, and dehydration may develop.

The composition of intracellular and extracellular fluids is an important factor in homeostasis. These fluids must have the proper levels of electrolytes and must be kept at a constant pH. The kidneys are the main regulators of body fluids. Other factors that aid in regulation include hormones, buffers, and respiration. The normal pH of body fluids is a slightly alkaline 7.4. When regulating mechanisms fail to control shifts in pH, either *acidosis* or *alkalosis* results.

Fluid therapy is used to correct fluid and electrolyte imbalances and to give a patient nourishment.

II. Topics for Review

A. Fluid compartments
   1. Intracellular fluid compartment
   2. Extracellular fluid compartment
      a. Special compartments
B. Water balance
   1. Intake
   2. Output
   3. Thirst center
C. Electrolytes
   1. Cations and anions
   2. Electrolyte balance
      a. Role of hormones
D. Acid–base balance (pH)
   1. Buffers
   2. Kidney function
   3. Respiration
E. Disorders of body fluids
F. Fluid therapy

III. Matching Exercises

Matching only within each group, write the answers in the spaces provided.

Group A

electrolyte   extracellular   buffer
normal saline   hydrogen ion   dextrose
intracellular

1. Term that describes fluids in spaces outside the body cells   _____

2. A compound that forms ions in solution   _____

3. Substance that determines the acidity or alkalinity of a fluid   _____

4. An isotonic solution that is often given in emergencies   _____

5. Term that describes the fluid within the body cells   _____

6. The sugar usually contained in nutritional fluids   _____

7. A substance that aids in maintaining a constant pH   _____

Group B

carbonic acid   homeostasis   diffusion
blood plasma   water   hypothalamus
edema

1. The substance that makes up 50% to 70% of a person's
    body weight   _____

2. The substance formed when carbon dioxide goes into
    solution in body fluids   _____

3. A portion of the extracellular fluid   _____

4. The process that allows constant interchanges to occur
    between fluid compartments   _____

5. A constancy of internal conditions, such as the
    composition of body fluids   _____

6. The part of the brain that controls the sense of thirst   _____

7. The presence of excessive fluid in the tissues   _____

Group C

alkalosis   cation   interstitial
dehydration   parathyroid hormone aldosterone
anion   ascites

1. A collection of fluid within the abdominal cavity   _____

2. An ion with a positive electrical charge

_____

3. Term that describes fluid located in the microscopic spaces between cells

_____

4. The adrenal hormone that promotes the reabsorption of sodium

_____

5. The term used to describe a serious fluid deficit

_____

6. An ion with a negative electrical charge

_____

7. A hormone that causes the kidney to reabsorb calcium

_____

8. An increase in the pH of body fluids, such as may result from hyperventilation

_____

IV. Multiple Choice

Select the best answer and write the letter of your choice in the blank.

1. Which of the following fluids is *not* in the extracellular compartment?

    a. blood plasma
    b. interstitial fluid
    c. cytoplasm
    d. cerebrospinal fluid
    e. lymph

    1. _____

2. Which of the following is *not* a route for water loss?

    a. synovial fluid
    b. urine
    c. exhaled air
    d. skin
    e. feces

    2. _____

3. Addison's disease is due to a deficiency of

    a. testosterone
    b. sex hormone
    c. DNA
    d. aldosterone
    e. potassium

    3. _____

4. Which of the following is *not* a potential cause of edema?

    a. protein deficiency
    b. congestive heart failure
    c. allergy
    d. lymphatic blockage
    e. dehydration

    4. _____

5. Polydipsia is

    a. loss of fluid
    b. excessive thirst
    c. excess sodium in the blood
    d. dehydration
    e. collection of fluid

5. _____

6. Aldosterone is produced by the

    a. pituitary
    b. adrenal medulla
    c. thymus
    d. adrenal cortex
    e. hypothalamus

6. _____

V. Labeling

For the following illustration, write the name or names of each labeled part on the numbered lines.

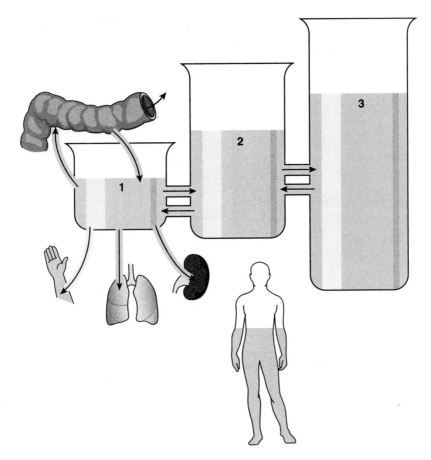

Main fluid compartments

1. _____   3. _____

2. _____

310

VI. True–False

For each question, write T for true or F for false in the blank to the left of each number. If a statement is false, correct it by replacing the underlined term and write the correct statement in the blanks below the question.

_____ 1. A substance with a pH below 7.0 is underlined alkaline.

_____

_____

_____ 2. A solution with a higher concentration than the fluid in the cell is termed hypotonic.

_____

_____

_____ 3. A solution of pH 4.0 is more acidic than a solution of pH 6.0.

_____

_____

_____ 4. Sodium and potassium ions are positively charged and, thus, are described as anions.

_____

_____

_____ 5. Body fluids are slightly alkaline.

_____

_____

_____ 6. The exhalation of carbon dioxide makes the blood more acidic.

_____

_____

VII. Completion Exercise

Write the word or phrase that correctly completes each sentence.

1. Water balance is partly regulated by a thirst center located in a region of the brain called the

_____

2. Blood plasma, interstitial fluid, and lymph are contained in the fluid compartment outside the cells. This compartment is described as the

_____

3. The normal pH of body fluids is

_____

4. The pH scale measures the concentration of

_____

5. A drop in pH of body fluids produces a condition called

_____

6. Accumulation of excessive fluid in the intercellular spaces is

_____

7. A fluid that has the same concentration as body fluids is described as

_____

VIII. Practical Applications

Study each discussion. Then write the appropriate word or phrase in the space provided.

1. Mr. B, age 38, had been traveling in Asia. He became ill with diarrhea, vomiting, and other symptoms of cholera. On admission to a hospital in the United States, he was found to be suffering from a severe fluid deficit, a condition called

_____

2. Mrs. G, age 62, complained of swelling of her lower extremities. She suffered from kidney failure, which caused an excessive accumulation of fluids in the tissues, a condition called

_____

3. Mr. K had been an alcoholic for several years. Now, he is suffering from liver disease and swelling of the abdomen due to an accumulation of fluid in the abdomen. This is called

_____

4. Mr. F had suffered from rheumatoid arthritis for several years. Now, he came in with symptoms of heart failure. X-ray studies showed a collection of fluid in the pericardial sac. Such a collection is called a(n)

_____

5. Mrs. G, age 38, had a known case of damage to the mitral valve, preventing the return of blood to the heart. At this time, she presented with shortness of breath and a cough with pink, foamy sputum. This serious disorder of body fluids, resulting from a backup of fluid in the lungs, is known as

_____

6. Jane had large areas of second- and third-degree burns. Edema of the burned areas was caused by damage to the smallest of the blood vessels, called

_____

IX. Short Essays

1. Briefly describe the control center for the sense of thirst.

   _____

   _____

   _____

2. Compare acidosis and alkalosis, and cite some causes of each.

   _____

   _____

   _____

3. Describe some circumstances under which fluid therapy might be given and cite some fluids that are used.

   _____

   _____

   _____

The Urinary System

I. Overview

The urinary system comprises two *kidneys,* two *ureters,* one *urinary bladder,* and one *urethra.* This system is thought of as the body's main excretory mechanism; it is, in fact, often called the *excretory system.* The kidney, however, performs other essential functions; it aids in maintaining water and electrolyte balance and in regulating the acid–base balance (pH) of body fluids. The kidneys also secrete a hormone that stimulates red blood cell production and an enzyme that acts to increase blood pressure.

The functional unit of the kidney is the *nephron.* It is the nephron that produces *urine* from substances filtered out of the blood through a cluster of capillaries, the *glomerulus.* The processes involved in urine formation in addition to filtration are tubular reabsorption, tubular secretion, and concentration of urine. Oxygenated blood is brought to the kidney by the *renal artery.* The arterial system branches through the kidney until the smallest subdivision, the *afferent arteriole,* carries blood into the glomerulus. Blood leaves the glomerulus by means of the *efferent arteriole* and eventually leaves the kidney by means of the *renal vein.* Before blood enters the venous network of the kidney, exchanges occur between the filtrate and the blood through the *peritubular capillaries* that surround each nephron.

Prolonged or serious diseases of the kidney have devastating effects on overall body function and health. Renal dialysis and kidney transplantation are effective methods for saving lives of people who otherwise would die of kidney failure and uremia.

II. Topics for Review

III. Matching Exercises

Matching only within each group, write the answers in the spaces provided.

Group A

Bowman's capsule	medulla	excretion
nephron	adipose capsule	fibrous capsule
retroperitoneal space	urine	

1. The process of removing waste products from the body _____

2. A microscopic functional unit of the kidney _____

3. The crescent of fat that helps to support the kidney _____

4. The fluid eliminated by the excretory system _____

5. The area behind the peritoneum that contains the ureters and the kidneys _____

6. A hollow bulb at the proximal end of the nephron _____

7. The membranous connective tissue that encloses the kidney _____

8. The inner region of the kidney _____

Group B

urea	glomerulus	filtration
renal pelvis	convoluted tubule	cortex
collecting ducts	epithelium	tubular reabsorption

1. The main tissue that makes up the kidney _____

2. The outer region of the kidney _____

3. The main nitrogenous waste product of the body _____

4. A coiled portion of a nephron _____

5. The process that returns useful substances in the filtrate to the bloodstream _____

6. The cluster of capillaries within Bowman's capsule of the nephron _____

7. The process by which substances leave the glomerulus and enter Bowman's capsule _____

8. The funnel-shaped basin that forms the upper end of the ureter _____

9. The tubes that receive urine from the distal convoluted tubules of the nephrons

    _____

Group C

urethra	micturition	electrolytes
hilus	calyces	glucose
peristalsis	protein	

1. The cuplike extensions of the renal pelvis that collect urine

    _____

2. The tube that carries urine from the bladder to the outside

    _____

3. The type of nutrient that always contains nitrogen

    _____

4. The rhythmic contractions that move urine along the ureter from the kidneys to the bladder

    _____

5. The area where the renal artery, renal vein, and ureter connect with the kidney

    _____

6. The simple sugar that appears in the urine in cases of diabetes mellitus

    _____

7. Another name for urination

    _____

8. Compounds that are normally contained in urine

    _____

Group D

uremia	hydrogen ion	cystitis
diffusion	pyelonephritis	pyramids
edema	renin	

1. Inflammation of the urinary bladder

    _____

2. Excessive accumulation of fluid in the body tissues, as may be caused by kidney failure

    _____

3. The process by which nitrogenous waste products are removed from the blood in dialysis

    _____

4. The enzyme produced by the kidney that acts to increase blood pressure

    _____

5. The substance that is adjusted by the kidney to regulate the pH of body fluids

    _____

6. Cone-shaped structures in the kidney medulla that contain tubules

    _____

7. Inflammation of the renal pelvis and the kidney tissue itself

    _____

8. The general condition caused by accumulation of nitrogenous waste products in the blood

    _____

Group E

polyuria	calculi	juxtaglomerular apparatus
specific gravity	trigone	tubular secretion
nocturia	erythropoietin	

1. Elimination of very large amounts of urine   _____

2. The process by which the renal tubule actively moves substances from the blood into the nephron to be excreted   _____

3. An indication of the amount of dissolved substances in the urine   _____

4. Kidney stones; solids formed when uric acid or calcium salts precipitate out of the urine instead of remaining in solution   _____

5. The structure in the kidney that produces renin   _____

6. The triangle at the base of the bladder   _____

7. The hormone released by the kidney that stimulates the bone marrow to produce red blood cells   _____

8. Elimination of urine during the night   _____

IV. Multiple Choice

Select the best answer and write the letter of your choice in the blank.

1. Which of the following is *not* a function of the kidneys?   1. _____

   a. adjust the composition of body fluids
   b. help regulate blood pressure
   c. regulate the volume of body fluids
   d. eliminate waste
   e. destroy red blood cells

2. Select the correct order of urine flow from its source to the outside of the body.   2. _____

   a. bladder, renal pelvis, urethra, ureter
   b. kidney, ureter, bladder, urethra
   c. urethra, bladder, kidney, ureter
   d. bladder, ureter, cortex, nephron
   e. renal pelvis, nephron, urethra, calyx

3. The urinary meatus is the   3. _____

   a. muscle in the wall of the bladder
   b. capillary bed around the loop of Henle
   c. external opening of the urethra
   d. valve around the ureter
   e. muscle around the urethra

4. The juxtaglomerular apparatus consists of cells in the   4. _____

     a. glomerulus and Bowman's capsule
     b. proximal convoluted tubule and efferent arteriole
     c. renal artery and cortex
     d. collecting tubules and renal vein
     e. distal convoluted tubule and afferent arteriole

5. The distal convoluted tubule is between   5. _____

     a. the collecting duct and calyx
     b. Bowman's capsule and the glomerulus
     c. the loop of Henle and the peritubular capillaries
     d. the loop of Henle and the collecting duct
     e. the proximal convoluted tubule and the renal vein

6. The enzyme renin raises blood pressure by activating   6. _____

     a. red blood cells
     b. glomerular filtrate
     c. angiotensin
     d. erythropoietin
     e. sodium

7. Which of the following is a normal constituent of urine?   7. _____

     a. albumin
     b. glucose
     c. casts
     d. urea
     e. blood

8. Kidney stones that are large enough to fill the kidney pelvis and extend into the calyces are called   8. _____

     a. polycystic kidneys
     b. staghorn calculi
     c. ptosis
     d. renal colic
     e. sphincters

9. The last part of each ureter enters at an angle through the lower bladder wall. This prevents   9. _____

     a. reabsorption
     b. concentration of urine
     c. backflow of urine
     d. glomerular filtration
     e. micturition

10. The congenital anomaly in which the urethra opens on the undersurface of the penis is known as   10. _____

     a. hypospadias
     b. glomerulonephritis
     c. hydronephrosis
     d. hypertension
     e. lithiasis

V. Labeling

For each of the following illustrations, write the name or names of each labeled part on the numbered lines.

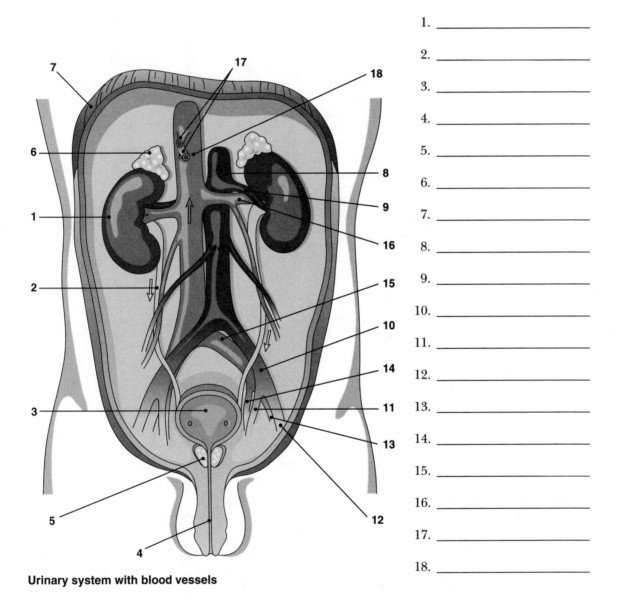

Urinary system with blood vessels

1. _____
2. _____
3. _____
4. _____
5. _____
6. _____
7. _____
8. _____
9. _____
10. _____
11. _____
12. _____
13. _____
14. _____
15. _____
16. _____
17. _____
18. _____

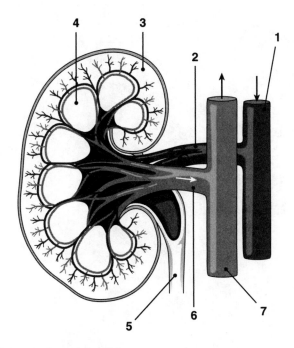

Blood supply and circulation of the kidney

1. _____

2. _____

3. _____

4. _____

5. _____

6. _____

7. _____

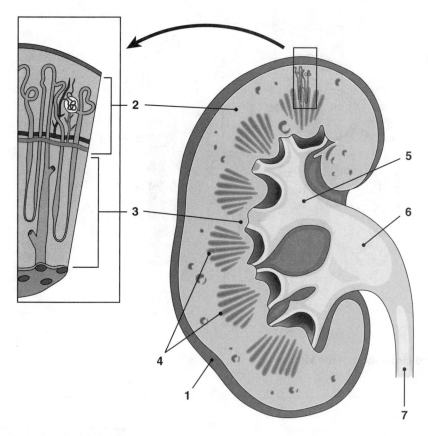

Longitudinal section through kidney

1. _____

2. _____

3. _____

4. _____

5. _____

6. _____

7. _____

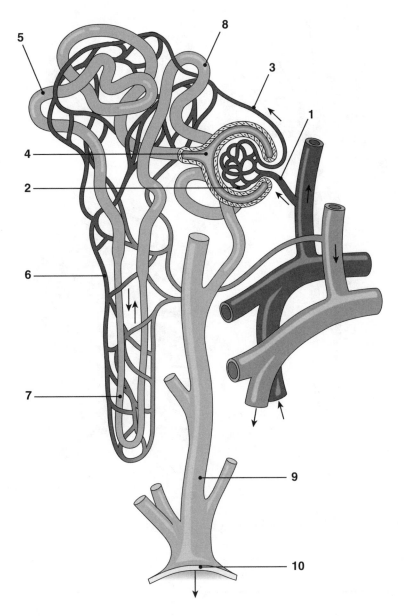

Simplified diagram of a nephron

1. _____   6. _____

2. _____   7. _____

3. _____   8. _____

4. _____   9. _____

5. _____   10. _____

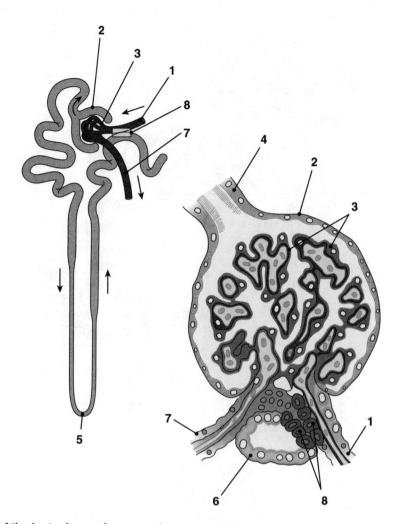

Structure of the juxtaglomerular apparatus

1. _____ 5. _____

2. _____ 6. _____

3. _____ 7. _____

4. _____ 8. _____

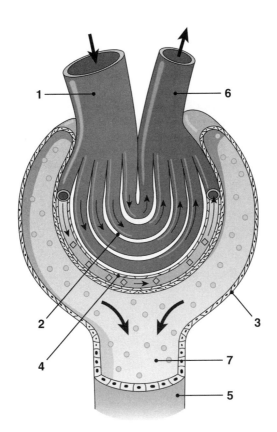

Process of filtration in the formation of urine

1. _____   5. _____

2. _____   6. _____

3. _____   7. _____

4. _____

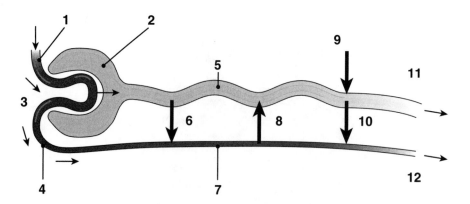

Summary of urine formation

1. _____   7. _____

2. _____   8. _____

3. _____   9. _____

4. _____   10. _____

5. _____   11. _____

6. _____   12. _____

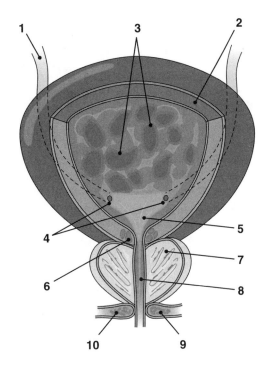

Interior of the urinary bladder

1. _____

2. _____

3. _____

4. _____

5. _____

6. _____

7. _____

8. _____

9. _____

10. _____

VI. True–False

For each question, write T for true or F for false in the blank to the left of each number. If a statement is false, correct it by replacing the underlined term and write the correct statement in the blanks below the question.

_____ 1. The outer portion of the kidney is the <u>medulla.</u>

_____ 2. Cystitis is inflammation of the <u>kidney.</u>

_____ 3. Glomerular filtrate flows from Bowman's capsule into the <u>proximal convoluted tubule.</u>

_____ 4. The <u>efferent arteriole</u> carries blood into the glomerulus.

_____ 5. Under the effects of ADH, water is <u>reabsorbed.</u>

_____ 6. The <u>urethra</u> transports urine from the kidney to the bladder.

_____ 7. Urine with a specific gravity of 0.04 is <u>more</u> concentrated than urine with a specific gravity of 0.02.

_____ 8. Angiotensin causes blood vessels to <u>constrict.</u>

_____ 9. The internal urethral sphincter is <u>involuntary.</u>

_____

_____

VII. Completion Exercise

Write the word or phrase that correctly completes each sentence.

1. There are many causes of ureteral obstruction. One of
   these is a kinking of the ureter that is due to a dropping
   of the kidney, or   _____

2. When the bladder is empty, its lining is thrown into the
   folds known as   _____

3. The vessel that carries oxygenated blood to the kidney is the   _____

4. A laboratory study of urine is called a(n)   _____

5. The straddle type of injury occurs when, for example, a man
   is walking along a raised beam and slips so that the beam is
   between his legs. Such an accident may rupture the duct that
   transports urine away from the bladder. This duct is the   _____

6. An important sign of urinary tract disease or injury is blood
   in the urine, a condition that is called   _____

7. In diabetes, starvation, and other conditions, fats are not
   completely oxidized. As a result, a test of the urine may
   reveal the presence of   _____

8. One indication of nephritis is the presence in the urine of
   molds that have been formed in the kidney tubules. They
   are called   _____

9. Diabetes insipidus is marked by great thirst and the
   elimination of large amounts of very dilute urine. The disease
   is caused by a lack of a hormone from the pituitary that
   regulates water reabsorption in the kidney. This hormone is   _____

VIII. Practical Applications

Study each discussion. Then write the appropriate word or phrase in the space
provided.

Group A

1. K, age 7, was brought to the clinic because his mother noted
   that his urine had a red hue. He had been quite ill with a
   "strep throat" a few weeks earlier. Tests indicated that K
   was suffering from the most common disease of the
   kidneys, namely   _____

2. K's mother, Mrs. L, age 31, was concerned because she had had several similar episodes during her childhood. She was assured that her son would recover with appropriate treatment and was advised to have her own urine tested. The tests demonstrated protein in her urine, indicating continuing damage to the kidney tubules. The presence of protein in the urine is called

_____

3. The x-ray examination of Ms. G's urinary tract revealed a structural abnormality of the ureter in the form of extreme narrowing, or

_____

4. Mrs. M was suffering from cystitis, a bladder infection. Studies indicated that there was relaxation of the pelvic floor, causing stagnation of urine in the bladder, and corrective surgery was planned. In preparation for this, a catheter was inserted into the external opening, the

_____

5. Mr. K, age 61, required several studies to determine the cause of obstruction of his urinary tract. Pus cells were found in his urine specimen, indicating an infection. The presence of pus in the urine is termed

_____

6. One of the studies done in Mr. K's case revealed an obstruction at the bladder neck, a disorder that is fairly common in men of his age. The obstruction was caused by enlargement of the gland through which the first part of the urethra passes. This gland is the

_____

Group B

1. Mr. R had been exposed to poisonous arsenic compounds in the chemical manufacturing plant where he was employed. He was suffering from an acute renal failure. To remove the accumulated nitrogenous waste products from his blood, Mr. R was treated by a diffusion process called

_____

2. Mrs. C, age 38, was hospitalized with serious illness and multiple disorders of blood chemistries. Her history included several episodes of kidney infection with inflammation of the glomeruli. Due to extensive damage and poor function of the kidneys, one of the treatment options considered was an operation in which the kidney of a healthy donor is implanted in a person with renal failure. This operation is called

_____

3. Mr. G, age 58, had not consulted a physician in many years. He was now admitted to the hospital seriously ill with many symptoms of renal failure. Despite aggressive treatment, Mr. G slipped into a coma. Ultrasound studies showed enlarged kidneys and ureters as the cause of his kidney damage. This disorder in which obstruction to urine flow damages kidney tissue is named

_____

4. Mr. M was seen for a checkup, at which time a routine
urinalysis showed the presence of glucose and ketones.
The finding of these abnormal constituents in the urine
is often an indication of the endocrine disorder known as _____

IX. Short Essays

1. Name three systems other than the urinary system that excrete wastes.
Specify the type of waste excreted by each.

_____

_____

_____

2. Explain the structure and action of the juxtaglomerular apparatus.

_____

_____

_____

3. Because the kidneys regulate the composition of body fluids, chronic renal
failure can lead to a number of disorders. Describe some of the problems
associated with chronic renal failure.

_____

_____

_____

Unit VII

PERPETUATING LIFE

Chapter

23

The Male and Female Reproductive Systems

I. Overview

Reproduction is the process by which life continues. Human reproduction is *sexual*, that is, it requires the union of two different *germ cells* or *gametes*. (Some simple forms of life can reproduce without a partner in the process of *asexual* reproduction.) These germ cells, the *spermatozoon* in males and the *ovum* in females, are formed by *meiosis*, a type of cell division in which the chromosome number is reduced to one half. When fertilization occurs and the gametes combine, the original chromosome number is restored.

The reproductive glands or *gonads* manufacture the gametes and also produce hormones. These activities are continuous in the male but cyclic in the female. The male gonad is the *testis*. The remainder of the male reproductive tract consists of passageways for storage and transport of spermatozoa; the male organ of copulation, the *penis;* and several glands that contribute to the production of *semen.*

The female gonad is the *ovary.* The ovum released each month at the time of *ovulation* travels through the *oviducts* to the *uterus,* where the egg, if fertilized, develops. If no fertilization occurs, the ovum, along with the built-up lining of the uterus, is eliminated through the *vagina* as the *menstrual flow.*

Reproduction is under the control of hormones from the *anterior pituitary,* which, in turn, is controlled by the *hypothalamus* of the brain. These organs respond to *feedback* mechanisms, which maintain proper hormone levels.

Aging causes changes in both the male and female reproductive systems. A gradual decrease in male hormone production begins as early as age 20 and continues throughout life. In the female, a more sudden decrease in activity occurs between ages 45 and 55 and ends in *menopause,* the cessation of menstruation and of the childbearing years.

II. Topics for Review

III. Matching Exercises

Matching only within each group, write the answers in the spaces provided.

Group A

ovum	prepuce	testosterone
epididymis	scrotum	seminiferous tubules
testis	spermatozoon	ovary

1. The male gonad   _____

2. The male hormone secreted by the interstitial cells
   of the testis   _____

3. The germ cell of the female   _____

4. The female gonad   _____

5. The sac suspended between the thighs that holds the testis _____

6. The germ cell of the male   _____

7. The coiled tube in which spermatozoa are stored as
   they mature and become motile   _____

8. The foreskin   _____

9. The coiled ducts in which germ cells develop in the testes _____

Group B

semen	gonad	acrosome
ejaculatory duct	gamete	urethra
spermatic cord	ductus deferens	seminal vesicles
FSH		

1. The general term for a sex gland   _____

2. The two glands located behind the urinary bladder
   in the male that contribute a large volume of the semen   _____

3. A caplike covering over the head of the spermatozoon
   that aids in penetration of the ovum   _____

4. The structure containing the ductus deferens, nerves,
   blood vessels, and lymphatic vessels that extends from
   the testis   _____

5. A male or female germ cell   _____

6. The hormone that stimulates Sertoli cells in the testis   _____

7. The tube formed by the union of the ductus deferens
   and the duct from the seminal vesicle   _____

8. In males, the single tube that conveys urine and semen to the outside

_____

9. The tube that extends upward from the epididymis and transports spermatozoa

_____

10. The mixture of spermatozoa and glandular secretions that is expelled in ejaculation

_____

Group C

phimosis	inguinal canal	gonorrhea
ejaculation	cryptorchidism	prostate
infertility	penis	oligospermia
vasectomy		

1. A series of muscular contractions by which semen is expelled

_____

2. In both males and females, a significantly lower than normal ability to reproduce

_____

3. The condition that results when the testes fail to descend into the scrotal sac during fetal life

_____

4. Tightness of the foreskin, which prevents it from being drawn back

_____

5. The gland that contributes to semen and is located below the urinary bladder in the male

_____

6. A deficiency in the number of sperm cells in the semen

_____

7. The channel through which the testis descends before birth

_____

8. A procedure for sterilizing a male by removing a portion of the ductus deferens, thus preventing spermatozoa from reaching the urethra

_____

9. A common sexually transmitted disease accompanied by burning and pain on urination and a discharge from the urethra in the male

_____

10. The organ that holds the longest part of the urethra in the male

_____

Group D

vulva	ovulation	vagina
fallopian tube	ovarian follicle	fimbriae
hymen	broad ligaments	uterus

1. An alternate name for the oviduct

_____

2. The muscular tube that serves as a birth canal

_____

3. Peritoneal structures that serve as anchors for the uterus and ovaries

_____

4. A fold of membrane found at the opening of the vagina

_____

5. A sac within which the ovum matures

_____

6. The muscular organ in which a fetus develops

_____

7. Fringelike extensions that sweep the ovum into the oviduct

_____

8. Discharge of an ovum from the surface of the ovary

_____

9. The external parts of the female reproductive system, consisting of the labia, the clitoris, and related structures

_____

Group E

dysmenorrhea	fundus	corpus
fornix	myoma	endometrium
amenorrhea	corpus luteum	cervix
salpingitis		

1. The main part, or body, of the uterus

_____

2. The circular recess formed as the uterus dips into the upper vagina

_____

3. Another term for a uterine growth known as a fibroid

_____

4. The small, rounded part of the uterus located above the openings of the oviducts

_____

5. The structure formed by the ruptured follicle after ovulation

_____

6. Painful or difficult menstruation

_____

7. The necklike part of the uterus that dips into the upper vagina

_____

8. Inflammatory infection of the oviducts

_____

9. The specialized tissue that lines the uterus

_____

10. Absence of the menstrual flow

_____

Group F

clitoris	menopause	mastectomy
estrogen	menses	luteinizing hormone
posterior fornix	follicle-stimulating hormone	hysterectomy

1. Cessation of reproductive activity in the female _____

2. A hormone from the pituitary that causes the ovum to develop _____

3. A small, highly sensitive organ in the vulva of the female _____

4. The dorsal space behind the upper vaginal canal that lies next to the deepest part of the peritoneal cavity in the female _____

5. A hormone from the pituitary that causes rupture of the ovarian follicle and release of the ovum midway during the menstrual cycle _____

6. Surgical removal of the breast _____

7. The ovarian hormone that begins the thickening of the endometrium early in the menstrual cycle _____

8. Surgical removal of the uterus _____

9. The menstrual flow _____

IV. Multiple Choice

Select the best answer and write the letter of your choice in the blank.

1. The glans penis is formed from the   1. _____

   a. pubic symphysis
   b. corpus cavernosum
   c. central artery
   d. corpus spongiosum
   e. interstitial cells

2. The hormones produced by the ovaries are   2. _____

   a. estrogen and progesterone
   b. oxytocin and FSH
   c. LH and testosterone
   d. ICSH and estrogen
   e. prolactin and progesterone

3. Which of the following is *not* part of the uterus?   3. _____

   a. fundus
   b. cervix
   c. fimbriae
   d. endometrium
   e. corpus

4. The most common cancer of the male reproductive system is cancer of the

   a. prostate
   b. testis
   c. epididymis
   d. urethra
   e. seminal vesicle

4. _____

5. The Pap smear is a test for

   a. ovarian cancer
   b. pregnancy
   c. cervical cancer
   d. breast cancer
   e. infertility

5. _____

6. A tubal ligation is done to

   a. remove the uterus
   b. promote fertilization
   c. sterilize a male
   d. sterilize a female
   e. increase sperm count

6. _____

7. Pelvic inflammatory disease is commonly caused by gonorrhea and by

   a. rickettsia
   b. chlamydia
   c. papillomavirus
   d. staphylococcus
   e. rubella

7. _____

8. The cul-de-sac is also called the

   a. fallopian tube
   b. uterosacral ligament
   c. labium majus
   d. retroperitoneal space
   e. rectouterine pouch

8. _____

9. The pelvic floor in both males and females is called the

   a. cervix
   b. fornix
   c. epididymis
   d. perineum
   e. acrosome

9. _____

10. Bartholin's glands are also called the

    a. greater vestibular glands
    b. labium minus
    c. obstetrical perineum
    d. bulbourethral glands
    e. Cowper's glands

10. _____

V. Labeling

For each of the following illustrations, write the name or names of each labeled part on the numbered lines.

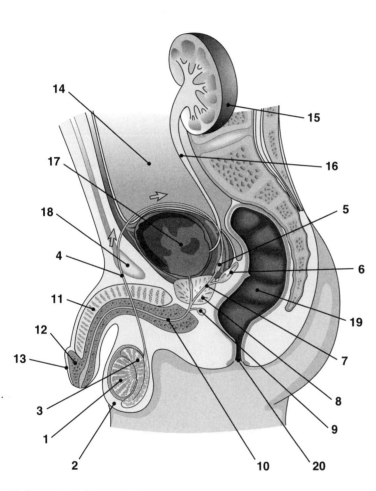

Male genitourinary system

1. _____

2. _____

3. _____

4. _____

5. _____

6. _____

7. _____

8. _____

9. _____

10. _____

11. _____

12. _____

13. _____

14. _____

15. _____

16. _____

17. _____

18. _____

19. _____

20. _____

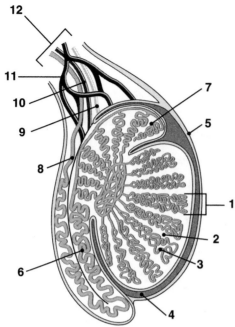

Structure of the testis

1. _____
2. _____
3. _____
4. _____
5. _____
6. _____
7. _____
8. _____
9. _____
10. _____
11. _____
12. _____

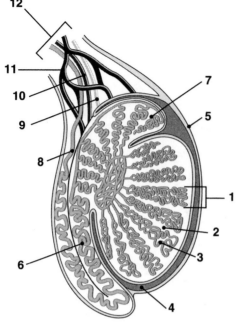

Cross section of the penis

1. _____
2. _____
3. _____
4. _____
5. _____
6. _____
7. _____
8. _____
9. _____
10. _____

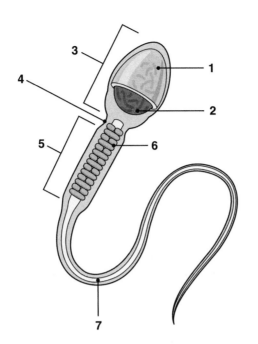

Human spermatozoon

1. _____

2. _____

3. _____

4. _____

5. _____

6. _____

7. _____

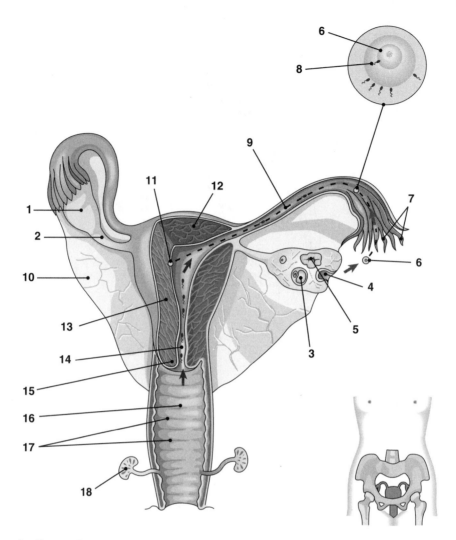

Female reproductive system

1. _____

2. _____

3. _____

4. _____

5. _____

6. _____

7. _____

8. _____

9. _____

10. _____

11. _____

12. _____

13. _____

14. _____

15. _____

16. _____

17. _____

18. _____

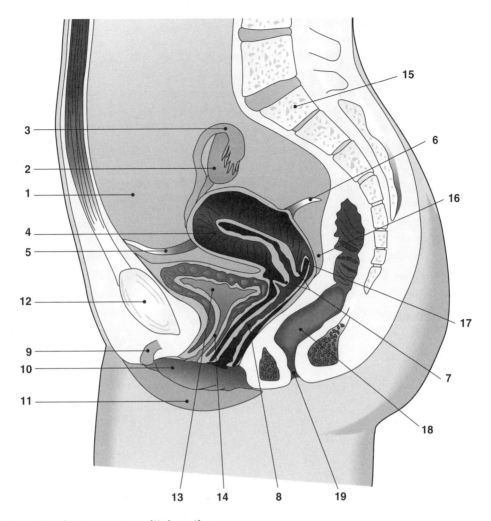

Female reproductive system, sagittal section

1. _____
2. _____
3. _____
4. _____
5. _____
6. _____
7. _____
8. _____
9. _____
10. _____

11. _____
12. _____
13. _____
14. _____
15. _____
16. _____
17. _____
18. _____
19. _____

1. _____

2. _____

3. _____

4. _____

5. _____

6. _____

7. _____

8. _____

9. _____

External female genitalia

VI. True–False

For each question, write T for true or F for false in the blank to the left of each number. If a statement is false, correct it by replacing the <u>underlined</u> term and write the correct statement in the blanks below the question.

_____ 1. The ductus deferens is also called the <u>vas deferens.</u>

_____

_____

_____ 2. Reproduction in simple life forms that requires no partner is described as <u>sexual.</u>

_____

_____

_____ 3. The interstitial cells of the testis secrete <u>hormones.</u>

_____

_____

_____ 4. The urethra is contained in the <u>corpus cavernosum</u> of the penis.

_____

_____

_____ 5. <u>Progesterone</u> is the first ovarian hormone produced in the menstrual cycle.

_____

_____

_____ 6. Painful or difficult menstruation is <u>amenorrhea.</u>

_____

_____

_____ 7. Luteinizing hormone in males is called <u>ICSH.</u>

_____

_____

VII. Completion Exercise

Write the word or phrase that correctly completes each sentence.

1. The process of cell division that reduces the chromosome number by half is _____

2. The region of the brain that controls the pituitary is the _____

3. The main male sex hormone is _____

4. The individual spermatozoon is very motile. It is able to move toward the ovum by the action of its _____

5. In the male, the tube that carries urine away from the bladder also carries sperm cells. This tube is the _____

6. In the region of the inguinal canal, the abdominal wall is somewhat weak. This weakness may allow abdominal organs to protrude through the wall, resulting in a condition known as _____

7. The testes are contained in an external sac called the _____

8. An x-ray study of the breasts for the detection of cancer is a(n) _____

9. The hormone that promotes development of spermatozoa in the male and development of an ovum in the female is _____

10. The use of artificial methods to prevent fertilization or implantation of the fertilized ovum is called _____

VIII. Practical Applications

Study each discussion. Then write the appropriate word or phrase in the space provided.

Group A

The following patients were seen by a physician in a urology clinic for men.

1. Mr. S, age 62, was referred by his physician because a rectal examination performed during his routine annual physical had revealed a nodule on his prostate gland. Further tests were required to determine whether the growth was benign or malignant. The studies were to include a blood test for PSA, which stands for _____

2. Mr. C, age 37, requested a surgical procedure that would render him sterile. This procedure, in which a segment of the ductus (vas) deferens is removed, is called a(n) _____

3. Mr. K, age 28, showed the doctor a number of fluid-filled vesicles (blisters) on his external genitals, and asked what they were. The doctor diagnosed a common sexually transmitted disease caused by a virus. This disease is called _____

4. Because Mr. K had not seen a physician for several years, a more complete examination was performed. Included was a blood test to determine whether he was suffering from a systemic sexually transmitted disease caused by a spirochete. This disorder occurs in three stages and is called _____

Group B

The following patients were seen by a physician in a clinic that specialized in women's health.

1. Mrs. K, age 43, thought that the bleeding she was now experiencing might be associated with early menopause. The physician examined her and found a firm mass in the upper part of the uterus. This might be a myoma, which is commonly called a(n) _____

2. Ms. C, age 26, was seen for a routine examination. A slide was made of the cells of the uterine cervix to be examined for cancer. This test is called a(n) _____

3. Mrs. J, age 47, came to the clinic with complaints of hot flashes and irregular bleeding. Her history included infrequent ovulation, as evidenced by her irregular menstrual cycles. The physician did a biopsy of the uterine lining as an aid in determining whether the bleeding was due to cancer. The lining of the uterus is the

_____

4. Janet was under treatment for a sexually transmitted chlamydial infection. Now, 2 days into her menstrual flow, she reported abdominal pain and a fever of 100.6°F. An ultrasound examination showed dilation of the ovarian tubes. To prevent further spread of the infection, Janet was to receive intravenous antibiotics. This generalized infection is abbreviated PID, which stands for

_____

IX. Short Essays

1. Describe the function of semen, and name the glands that contribute secretions to semen.

_____

_____

_____

2. Name the microorganisms that commonly cause infections of the reproductive tract in males and females.

_____

_____

_____

3. Define *contraception,* and describe how several common methods of contraception work.

_____

_____

_____

24

Development and Birth

I. Overview

Pregnancy begins with fertilization of an ovum by a spermatozoon to form a *zygote*. Over the next 38 weeks of *gestation*, the offspring develops first as an *embryo* and then as a *fetus*. During this period, it is nourished and maintained by the *placenta*, formed from tissues of both the mother and the embryo.

Childbirth or *parturition* occurs in four stages, beginning with contractions of the uterus and dilation of the cervix. Subsequent stages include delivery of the infant, delivery of the afterbirth, and control of bleeding.

Milk production, or *lactation,* is stimulated by the hormones prolactin and oxytocin from the pituitary gland. Removal of milk from the breasts is the stimulus for continued production.

II. Topics for Review

A. Pregnancy
   1. Fertilization
   2. Embryo
   3. Placenta
   4. Amniotic sac
   5. Fetus
B. Childbirth
   1. Stages
   2. Multiple births
C. Lactation
D. Disorders of pregnancy, delivery, and lactation

III. Matching Exercises

Matching only within each group, write the answers in the spaces provided.

Group A

placenta	ultrasonography	implantation
amniotic fluid	progesterone	perineum
embryo	gestation	puerperal

1. The pelvic floor in both males and females   _____

2. The hormone produced by the corpus luteum that
   prepares the endometrium for the fertilized ovum   _____

3. The period of development in the uterus   _____

4. Attachment of the fertilized egg to the lining of the uterus   _____

5. The flat, circular structure that serves as the organ for
   nutrition, respiration, and excretion for the fetus   _____

6. The substance that surrounds the developing offspring
   and serves as a protective cushion   _____

7. Method used to monitor pregnancy and delivery   _____

8. Term that means *related to childbirth*

_____

9. Term for the developing offspring from fertilization of an ovum until the third month of growth

_____

Group B

dilation   umbilicus   fetus
chorionic gonadotropin   afterbirth   parturition
lactation   prolactin

1. The scientific name for the navel

_____

2. The pituitary hormone that stimulates the secretion of milk by the mammary glands

_____

3. The process of giving birth to a child; labor

_____

4. The developing offspring from the third month until birth

_____

5. Widening of the opening of the cervix during labor

_____

6. The secretion of milk

_____

7. The placenta, together with the membranes of the amniotic sac and most of the umbilical cord, as they are expelled after delivery of a child

_____

8. A hormone produced by embryonic cells that maintains the corpus luteum early in pregnancy

_____

Group C

zygote   oxytocin   ectopic
embryology   mastitis   colostrum
vernix caseosa   abortion   umbilical cord

1. Inflammation of the breast

_____

2. The first mammary gland secretion to appear during lactation

_____

3. A fertilized egg

_____

4. Loss of a fetus before the 20th week of gestation

_____

5. The cheeselike material that protects the skin of the fetus

_____

6. The pituitary hormone that promotes the ejection of milk from the mammary glands

_____

7. The study of early development

_____

8. The structure that supplies nutrients and oxygen to the fetus and carries away waste

_____

9. Term for a pregnancy that develops outside the uterine cavity

_____

IV. Multiple Choice

Select the best answer and write the letter of your choice in the blank.

1. Edema, protein in the urine, and hypertension are all symptoms of a serious disorder of pregnancy known as

   1. _____

   a. preeclampsia
   b. placenta previa
   c. mastitis
   d. parturition
   e. amniocentesis

2. Fetal circulation is designed to bypass the

   2. _____

   a. heart
   b. lungs
   c. liver
   d. spleen
   e. brain

3. A surgical cut and repair of the perineum to prevent tearing of tissue during childbirth is a(n)

   3. _____

   a. hysterectomy
   b. mastectomy
   c. episiotomy
   d. eclampsia
   e. hernia

4. Premature separation of the placenta from the wall of the uterus is

   4. _____

   a. choriocarcinoma
   b. ectopic pregnancy
   c. placenta previa
   d. orchitis
   e. abruptio placentae

5. Twins that result from two different ova being fertilized by two different sperm cells are described as

   5. _____

   a. monozygotic
   b. identical
   c. fraternal
   d. preterm
   e. umbilical

6. The second stage of labor includes

    a. expulsion of the afterbirth
    b. the onset of contractions
    c. implantation of the embryo
    d. passage of the fetus through the vagina
    e. expulsion of the placenta

6. _____

7. The term *viable* is used to describe a fetus that is

    a. spontaneously aborted
    b. delivered by cesarean section
    c. developing outside the uterus
    d. capable of living outside the uterus
    e. stillborn

7. _____

V. Labeling

For each of the following illustrations, write the name or names of each labeled part on the numbered lines.

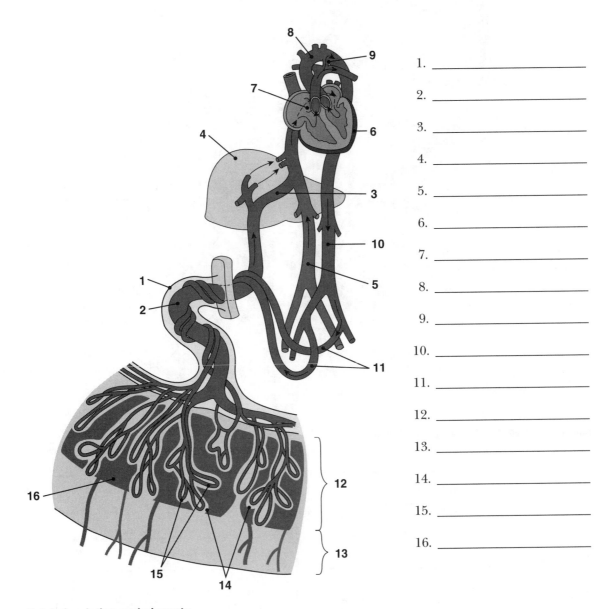

Fetal circulation and placenta

1. _____
2. _____
3. _____
4. _____
5. _____
6. _____
7. _____
8. _____
9. _____
10. _____
11. _____
12. _____
13. _____
14. _____
15. _____
16. _____

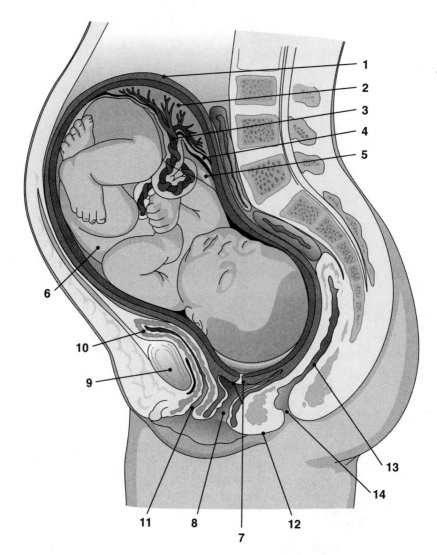

Midsagittal section of a pregnant uterus

1. _____
2. _____
3. _____
4. _____
5. _____
6. _____
7. _____

8. _____
9. _____
10. _____
11. _____
12. _____
13. _____
14. _____

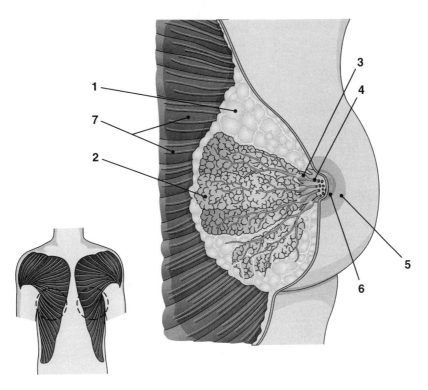

Section of the breast

1. _____   5. _____

2. _____   6. _____

3. _____   7. _____

4. _____

VI. True–False

For each question, write T for true or F for false in the blank to the left of each number. If a statement is false, correct it by replacing the underlined term and write the correct statement in the blanks below the question.

_____ 1. For the first 8 weeks of life in the uterus, the developing child is referred to as a <u>fetus.</u>

_____

_____

_____ 2. The beginnings of all body systems are established during the <u>first trimester.</u>

_____

_____

_____ 3. The afterbirth is expelled during the <u>third stage</u> of labor.

_____

_____

_____ 4. <u>Fraternal twins</u> develop from a single fertilized egg.

_____

_____

_____ 5. There are <u>two</u> umbilical arteries.

_____

_____

_____ 6. Blood is carried from the placenta to the fetus in the <u>umbilical vein</u>.

_____

_____

VII. Completion Exercise

Write the word or phrase that correctly completes each sentence.

1. By the end of the first month of embryonic life, the beginnings of the extremities may be seen. These are four small swellings called _____

2. The cell formed by the union of a male and a female gamete is called a(n) _____

3. The science that deals with the development of the embryo is called _____

4. The "bag of waters" is a popular name for the membranous sac that encloses the fetus. The scientific name for this structure is _____

5. The medical term for the loss of an embryo or fetus before the 20th week of pregnancy is _____

6. The mammary glands of the female provide nourishment for the newborn through the secretion of milk; this is a process called _____

7. An infant born before the organ systems are mature is considered immature or _____

8. The cutting of the perineum to reduce tearing during childbirth is called a(n) _____

VIII. Practical Applications

Study each discussion. Then write the appropriate word or phrase in the space provided.

1. Mrs. G complained of soreness and discomfort of the breasts after the birth of her baby. The physician diagnosed her disorder as inflammation of the breast, or _____

2. Because of episodes of hemorrhage during her pregnancy, Mrs. M was hospitalized. There was a possibility that in Mrs. M's case the placenta was attached to the lower part of the uterus instead of the upper part. This condition is known as _____

3. Because of the seriousness of Mrs. M's condition, an operation was considered; this would provide for delivery through an incision made in the abdominal wall and the wall of the uterus. This operation is called a(n) _____

4. Denise had missed several periods and suspected she was pregnant, but she did not consult a physician until her pregnancy was in its second trimester. The gestation period is 38 weeks, but if pregnancy is dated from the last menstrual period, its length is measured as _____

5. Denise's physician wanted to check for possible abnormalities and determine the age of her fetus. For this purpose, she used a technique for visualizing soft tissues without the use of x-rays. The form of energy used for this imaging technique is known as _____

IX. Short Essays

1. What is a puerperal infection, and how has the incidence of such infections changed over time?

   _____

   _____

   _____

2. What is a cesarean section, and why is it done?

   _____

   _____

   _____

3. Name the hormones that are involved in lactation, and describe what they do.

   _____

   _____

   _____

Heredity and Hereditary Diseases

I. Overview

The scientific study of heredity has advanced with amazing speed in the past 50 years. Nevertheless, many mysteries remain. Gregor Mendel was the first person known to have carried out formal experiments in genetics. He identified independent units of heredity, which he called *factors* and which we now call **genes**.

The chromosomes in the nucleus of each cell are composed of a complex molecule, **DNA**. This material makes up the many thousands of genes that determine a person's traits and are passed on to offspring at the time of fertilization. Genes direct the formation of **enzymes**, which, in turn, make possible all the chemical reactions of metabolism. Defective genes, produced by **mutation**, may disrupt normal enzyme activity and result in hereditary disorders such as sickle cell anemia, albinism, and phenylketonuria. Some human traits are determined by a single pair of genes (one gene from each parent), but most are controlled by multiple pairs of genes acting together.

Genes may be classified as **dominant** or **recessive.** If one parent contributes a dominant gene, then any offspring who receives that gene will show the trait (eg, Huntington's chorea). Traits carried by recessive genes may remain hidden for generations and be revealed only if they are contributed by both parents (eg, albinism, cystic fibrosis, PKU, and sickle cell anemia). In some cases, treatment begun early may help prevent problems associated with a genetic disorder. Genetic counseling should be sought by all potential parents whose relatives are known to have an inheritable disorder.

II. Topics for Review

III. Matching Exercises

Matching only within each group, write the answers in the spaces provided.

Group A

mutation	meiosis	carrier
chromosomes	congenital	genes
dominant		

1. The type of cell division that forms the gametes _____

2. Independent units of heredity _____

3. A change in the genetic material of a cell _____

4. Term that describes a condition that exists at birth _____

5. The threadlike bodies in the nucleus that contain the genes _____

6. Term that describes a gene that is always expressed if present _____

7. Term for a person who has a recessive gene that is not expressed _____

Group B

karyotype	enzyme	hereditary
XY	sex-linked	XX
DNA		

1. A protein that promotes a chemical reaction within a cell _____

2. Term for a trait carried on the X chromosome, such as hemophilia _____

3. The complex chemical that makes up the chromosomes _____

4. The sex chromosomes that appear in female cells _____

5. A study of the chromosomes, as done on fetal cells collected before birth _____

6. Term that describes traits transmitted by genes _____

7. The sex chromosomes that appear in male cells _____

Group C

osteogenesis imperfecta	multifactorial	amniocentesis
albinism	pedigree	mutagenic
familial	phenylketonuria	

1. An inherited disorder of metabolism that involves an amino acid _____

2. Term for an agent that is known to produce changes in the genetic material of cells   _____

3. A complete family history; a family tree   _____

4. Removal of fluid from the sac surrounding the fetus   _____

5. A word that means hereditary   _____

6. The form of inheritance in which traits are determined by two or more pairs of genes acting together   _____

7. A disease of brittle bones   _____

8. A hereditary condition in which there is a lack of skin and hair pigment   _____

IV. Multiple Choice

Select the best answer and write the letter of your choice in the blank.

1. The person who is credited with the first scientific study of heredity was an Austrian monk named   1. _____

   a. John Down
   b. Gregor Mendel
   c. Bernard Sachs
   d. Alexander Wilson
   e. H. F. Klinefelter

2. Genes act by controlling the manufacture of   2. _____

   a. enzymes
   b. sugars
   c. DNA
   d. mutagens
   e. oxygen

3. The hereditary disease PKU involves the metabolism of the amino acid   3. _____

   a. lysine
   b. arginine
   c. glycolipid
   d. phenylalanine
   e. asparagine

4. Klinefelter's syndrome is a   4. _____

   a. disorder in which masses grow along the nerves
   b. form of dwarfism
   c. metabolic disorder
   d. condition of having extra fingers
   e. disorder that involves the sex chromosomes

5. The name *karyotype* for the genetic test refers to the fact
   that the chromosomes of the cell are located in the

   a. membrane
   b. cytoplasm
   c. nucleus
   d. endoplasmic reticulum
   e. ribosomes

5. _____

V. True–False

For each question, write T for true or F for false in the blank to the left of each
number. If a statement is false, correct it by replacing the underlined term and
write the correct statement in the blanks below the question.

_____ 1. Sex-linked traits appear almost exclusively in females.

_____

_____

_____ 2. The Y chromosome is the larger of the two sex chromosomes.

_____

_____

_____ 3. The sex of the offspring is determined by the sex chromosome carried
          in the sperm.

_____

_____

_____ 4. Every cell in the body except the germ cells contains 46 chromosomes.

_____

_____

_____ 5. A gene that must be inherited from both parents to appear is described
          as dominant.

_____

_____

_____ 6. If a cell with 46 chromosomes divides by meiosis, each daughter cell
          will have 23 chromosomes.

_____

_____

VI. Completion Exercise

Write the word or phrase that correctly completes each sentence.

1. A gene that is always expressed when present is described as _____

2. A change in a gene or chromosome is called a(n) _____

3. A person who shows no evidence of a trait but can pass a gene for that trait to an offspring is a(n) _____

4. In the disorder phenylketonuria, the amino acid phenylalanine cannot be metabolized because a protein is lacking in the cells. This protein functions as a(n) _____

5. The inherited condition in which skin and hair are strikingly white is _____

6. The number of chromosomes in each human germ cell is _____

VII. Practical Applications

Study each discussion. Then write the appropriate word or phrase in the space provided.

Group A

These patients were seen in a pediatric clinic.

1. A rigid diet had been prescribed for infant M after it had been determined that he had an inherited disorder characterized by a lack of the enzyme required for metabolism of phenylalanine. Infant M's disorder is called _____

2. NS, a black child, age 9, was seen in clinic due to a sudden onset of swelling of the joints of his hands and feet. Hemoglobin studies showed an abnormal type of hemoglobin typical of a disorder in which the red cells become crescent-shaped and clog small blood vessels. This hereditary abnormality is known as _____

3. TS, a 6-year-old white child, had a history of difficulty in breathing, frequent respiratory infections, and a digestive disorder for which a pancreatic extract was prescribed. These problems are typical of a hereditary disorder found mostly in whites, namely _____

4. Baby D's face was round; her eyes were close-set and slanted upward at the sides. The infant's condition, which is usually due to a defect in a germ cell, is termed _____

5. Young Mrs. L brought in her 2-year-old son to check his response to his prescribed diet and thiamin supplements. In this child's hereditary disorder, the urine has such a peculiar odor that the disease is often called

_____

Group B

In a university clinic, studies of several hereditary disorders were underway. Read each discussion and respond in the space provided.

1. Mrs. Y, age 38, was pregnant a second time. Her first child had Down syndrome, and she was apprehensive that a second child would be similarly affected. A study of the fluid in the sac surrounding the embryo was ordered. This procedure is called a(n)

_____

2. The cells from Mrs. Y's amniotic fluid were grown (cultured) and then stained for special study. A diagnosis of Down syndrome was made, based on the presence of an extra

_____

3. Mrs. G and her husband received genetic counseling. They had one normal child and one with albinism. They wanted to know whether there was a possibility that a third child would also have this genetic disorder. Neither parent showed the trait, but they feared that they might be capable of passing the disorder to their children. A person who does not exhibit a disorder but can pass a gene for the disorder to offspring is described as a(n)

_____

4. Mr. H, age 25, was scheduled for a checkup and discussion of his diet and medication. He had a hereditary disorder, Wilson's disease, in which there is abnormal accumulation of the metallic ion

_____

5. Mr. H was warned by his physician that continued disregard of his dietary prescription and prescribed medication would lead to damage to the largest organ of the abdomen, namely the

_____

6. Mrs. G, age 26, had postponed starting a family because her grandfather had polycystic disease. Her mother, age 50, had no evidence of this disease, although a 40-year-old uncle also had the disorder. To help Mrs. G make a decision about family planning, the genetic counselor prepared a detailed family history, called a(n)

_____

VIII. Short Essays

1. Explain how a child can be born with a specific trait that neither parent has.

   _____

   _____

   _____

2. Some traits in a population show a range instead of two clearly alternate forms. List some of these traits, and explain what causes this variety.

   _____

   _____

   _____

3. What are some of the methods used by genetic counselors in advising prospective parents?

   _____

   _____

   _____

4. Define *mutagenic agent,* and give several examples.

   _____

   _____

   _____

26

Medical Terminology

I. Overview

Medical terminology is the special language used worldwide by people in health occupations. Many terms used today originated from Latin or Greek words, but some have come from more recent languages such as French and German. New words are being added constantly as discoveries are made and the need for words to describe them arises. Because scientific knowledge grows in different places at the same time, there may be two or even more terms in use that mean the same thing. Efforts are always being made, however, to standardize the terminology so that people all over the world will "speak the same language."

Not only does medical terminology have universal application, but there are other advantages to its use. Often someone will say, "Why not use simple plain English?" The fact is that often there is no common word that is as precise as the scientific term. Moreover, one word or perhaps two can do the work of several sentences in descriptive force and accuracy. Medical terminology is a kind of shorthand; health workers should be so familiar with it that it becomes a "second language" with which they feel completely at ease.

Most medical words are made up of two or more parts. The main part, to which the other parts are attached, is called the root. These other parts include prefixes, which come before the root, and suffixes, which follow the root. A combining form is a root with a vowel added to make pronunciation easier. If more than one root or combining form makes up the word, it is a compound word. Take the time to divide each medical word into its parts and then look up the meaning of each part, studying each as you go; you will soon add many words to your vocabulary. Then if you practice saying the word, you will feel at ease with medical terminology. Here are some examples:

1. *Hypothermia* (hi-po-THER-me-ah): below-normal body temperature, usually due to excessive exposure to cold weather or icy water
   a. prefix: *hypo* = below normal
   b. root: *therm* = heat
   c. suffix: *ia* = condition or state of being
2. *Cardiopulmonary* (kar-de-o-PUL-mo-nar-e): related to heart and lungs
   a. combining form: *cardio* = heart
   b. root: *pulmon* = related to the lungs
   c. suffix: *ary* = pertaining to
3. *endometritis* (en-do-me-TRI-tis): inflammation of the lining of the uterus
   a. prefix: *endo* = within
   b. root: *metr* = the uterus
   c. suffix: *itis* = inflammation
4. *abdominohysterectomy* (ab-dom-ih-no-his-ter-EK-to-me): removal of the uterus through the abdominal wall
   a. combining form: *abdomino* = belly or abdomen
   b. root: *hyster* = uterus or womb
   c. suffix: *ectomy* = removal of

II. Topics for Review

A. Common roots and combining forms, such as
   abdomin-, abdomino-
   aden-, adeno-
   arthr-, arthro-
   bio-
   carcin-, carcino-

cardi-, cardio-
cephal-, cephalo-
chol-, chole-
chondr-, chondro-
cleid-, cleido-
cost-
cyt-, cyto-
derm-, derma-
enter-, entero-
gastr-, gastro-
gyn-, gyne-, gyneco-
hem-, hema-, hemato-, hemo-
hist-, histo-, histio-
hyster-, hystero-
idio-
lact-, lacto-
leuc-, leuk-, leuko-
nephr-, nephro-
neur-, neuro-
phag-, phago-
psych-, psycho-
somat-, somato-
vas-, vaso-

B. Common prefixes (beginnings of words), such as
a-, an-
ab-
circum-
contra-
di-
ex-
infra-
inter-
intra-
macro-
mal-
meg-, mega-, megalo-
met-, meta-
micro-
neo-
semi-
sub-
trans-
tri-
uni-

C. Common suffixes (word endings), such as
-algia
-cele
-ectasis
-ectomy
-esthesia
-ferent
-gen

-geny
-gram
-graph
-itis
-logy
-oma
-penia
-plasty
-pnea
-ptosis
-stomy
-tomy

D. Common adjective endings, such as *-ous* and *-al*

E. Common noun endings including *-us* and *-um*

III. Matching Exercises

Matching only within each group, write the answers in the spaces provided.

Group A

prefix	suffix	root
-ous	-cele	a-
compound word	combining form	

1. The foundation of a word

    _____

2. A word ending used to change the meaning of the
    word root

    _____

3. An ending that indicates the adjective form

    _____

4. The part of a word that precedes its root and changes
    its meaning

    _____

5. A word that contains two or more word roots or
    combining forms

    _____

6. A word root followed by a vowel to make pronunciation
    easier

    _____

7. A prefix that denotes absence or deficiency

    _____

8. A suffix that means a swelling or an enlarged space

    _____

Group B

psych-	hema-	somat-
cyt-	aden-	neo-
hist-	-algia	-sis
-graph		

1. A word part that means *blood*

    _____

2. A prefix that means *new* _____

3. A root that shows relation to a cell _____

4. A suffix that means *instrument for recording* _____

5. A root that means *gland* _____

6. A root that indicates the body _____

7. A suffix that means *condition* or *process* _____

8. A root that shows relation to the mind _____

9. A suffix that refers to pain _____

10. A root meaning *tissue* _____

Group C

arthr-	-itis	carcin-
-esthesia	infra-	-ptosis
meg-	-ectasis	-ectomy

1. A root that indicates a cancer _____

2. A prefix that indicates excessively large _____

3. A suffix that indicates inflammation _____

4. A word ending that indicates dilation or expansion of a part _____

5. A suffix that means *downward displacement* _____

6. A suffix that means *removal* or *destruction of a part* _____

7. A root that shows relation to a joint _____

8. A prefix that indicates that a part is located below _____

9. A suffix that refers to sensation _____

Group D

peri-	angio-	-tomy
leuko-	-genic	-penia
-stomy	erythr-	ab-
-ism		

1. A word part that means *red* _____

2. A suffix that means *a lack of* _____

3. A root that means *vessel* _____

4. A word part that means *white* _____

5. An ending that means *state of* _____

6. A prefix that means *around* _____

7. A suffix that indicates the formation of a new opening _____

8. A suffix that means *producing* _____

9. A prefix that means *away from* _____

10. A suffix that means *incision into a part* _____

Group E

Combine word parts from the list below to form words that match each of the following definitions. Write the correct words in the blanks.

hemo-, hemat-, hemato   aden-   -logy
-costal   oste-, osteo-   cyto-, -cyte
inter-   -lysis   carcin-
-ectomy   bio-   -cellular
-itis   -oma   intra-

1. The study of living things _____

2. Inflammation of bone _____

3. Removal of a gland _____

4. The scientific study of cells _____

5. Referring to the space between the ribs _____

6. A cancerous tumor _____

7. The study of blood and its constituents _____

8. A bone cell _____

9. A tumor filled with blood _____

10. The word that means *between cells* _____

11. A tumor made of glandular tissue _____

12. The dissolution or disintegration of blood cells (especially red blood cells) _____

13. The word that means inside of or within a cell _____

14. A firm tumor made of bone or bonelike tissue _____

15. Destruction or dissolution of body cells _____

Group F

Combine two or three word parts from the list below for a word that matches each of the following definitions. Write the appropriate words in the spaces provided.

electro-	micro-	cardio-
-graph	-gram	-centesis
-emia	arthro-	-esthesia
an-	encephalo-	-scope

1. Instrument for viewing small objects _____

2. A lack of red blood cells or hemoglobin _____

3. An x-ray image of the head (including the brain) _____

4. The instrument that is used for producing a graphic tracing of electric current in the heart muscle _____

5. Tapping or perforation of a joint _____

6. A lack of sensation (especially of pain) _____

7. A graphic record of electric currents in the brain (brain waves) _____

8. Instrument used to examine a joint _____

9. The instrument used for producing a graphic record of brain waves _____

10. The tracing of electric current in the heart muscle _____

11. Surgical perforation of the heart _____

IV. Completion Exercise

Write the word or phrase that correctly completes each sentence.

1. A prefix that indicates very small size is _____

2. Words that refer to an instrument for recording end with _____

3. The visible record produced by a recording instrument is indicated by a word ending in _____

4. A prefix that means *equal* or *the same* is _____

5. To show that something is outside or is sent outside, use the prefix _____

6. To indicate that there are three parts to an organ, begin the word with the prefix _____

7. A prefix that means *across, through,* or *beyond* is _____

8. To indicate surgical molding, use the suffix _____

9. The prefix that shows something is within the structure is _____

10. The noun form of the adjective *mucous* is _____

11. A root that means *to eat* or *to ingest* is _____

12. The suffix that means *bladder* or *sac* is _____

13. The prefix that means *away from* is _____

14. The suffix that means *painful* is _____

15. A suffix that means *removal by surgery or other means* is _____

16. A two-letter prefix that means *absence* or *lack of* is _____

17. A suffix that means *dilation* or *expansion* of a part is _____

18. A suffix that means *produced from* or *producing* is _____

19. The word root for tissue is _____

20. Prefixes that mean *excessively large* include _____

V. Practical Applications

Study each discussion. Then write the appropriate word or phrase in the space provided.

1. Mr. A, age 74, was evaluated in the family practice clinic because of weakness and inability to care for himself. The physician noted that Mr. A suffered from malnutrition. Later studies showed there was evidence of malunion of a fracture of the right thigh bone. The prefix *mal-* means _____

2. Baby John was brought to the clinic by his observant mother because one of his eyes did not seem normal. The doctor noted that there was unilateral enlargement of the right pupil and that this uniocular condition would require laboratory investigation. The prefix *uni-* means _____

3. Mrs. B was seen in urgent care for treatment of an injured hand. The physician noted that x-ray studies of the metacarpal bones showed possible fractures. The prefix *meta-* in *metacarpal* means

_____

4. Ms. C was examined in the outpatient department. It was noted that she had circumoral pallor and that this pallor was circumscribed. The prefix *circum-* means

_____

5. Later examination of Ms. C showed ptosis (TO-sis) of several abdominal organs, a condition called visceroptosis (vis-er-op-TO-sis). The word part *ptosis* may also be used as a separate word. It means

_____

6. Mrs. A was admitted for surgery because of bleeding from the uterus. One word root for uterus is *metr-;* another is

_____

7. A first-aid measure that everyone should be able to perform involves the heart and the lungs. This type of resuscitation is described by the compound word for heart and lungs, which is

_____